PSYCHIATRY - THEORY, APPLICATIONS AND TREATMENTS

A HOLISTIC CARE PROGRAM FOR PSYCHIATRIC REHABILITATION IN A CHINESE CONTEXT

PSYCHIATRY - THEORY, APPLICATIONS AND TREATMENTS

Additional books in this series can be found on Nova's website under the Series tab.

Additional e-books in this series can be found on Nova's website under the e-book tab.

PSYCHIATRY - THEORY, APPLICATIONS AND TREATMENTS

A HOLISTIC CARE PROGRAM FOR PSYCHIATRIC REHABILITATION IN A CHINESE CONTEXT

ANDREW LEUNG LUK

nova publishers
New York

For permission to use material from this book please contact us:
Telephone 631-231-7269; Fax 631-231-8175
Web Site: http://www.novapublishers.com

NOTICE TO THE READER

Library of Congress Cataloging-in-Publication Data

ISBN: 978-1-62618-004-8

Library of Congress Control Number: 2013931032

Published by Nova Science Publishers, Inc. † New York

CONTENTS

FOREWORD

Working as a frontline nurse for more than 13 years, I have encountered patients with different kinds of acute and chronic illnesses. They not only suffer from physical pain which leave them no choice but to seek for medical treatment, but also psychological distress triggered from their imbalance of health. Those patients with chronic illness which require social support may even lose hope and meaning of life, perceiving oneself as without any contribution to the society and a burden to their family members. Regarding patients with serious mental illness, they have a long way of rehabilitation and may easily be stigmatized. It is difficult for them to reintegrate into the society.

Upon the request of an ex-mental patient, a founder of the Christian Oi Hip Fellowship, a self-help group with a holistic care approach was established with the help of mental health professionals and hospital chaplains to offer an extra means to their rehabilitation. It is the intention of this book to describe the inception of the organization, the theory behind the holistic program, the intervention approach and the evidences found during more than 20 years of its development. It is hoped this book will arouse the awareness of healthcare professionals of the holistic needs of our clients, especially the spiritual dimension which is always neglected. Since I am in the nursing background and also study in the social work faculty, and the group counselors of the Fellowship are mostly psychiatric nurses and social workers, I would highlight the holistic care from the nursing and social work perspectives.

The content of this book is mainly based on my PhD thesis on "The changes of ex-mental patients attending a psychiatric rehabilitation program with holistic care". I would like to express my most sincere gratitude to all participants of the Christian Oi Hip Fellowship who shared their experiences in the self-help groups and that enriched our knowledge in this under-research area. I would also like to give my appreciation to Professor Daniel T. L. Shek, thesis supervisor, for his guidance, stimulation and encouragement during the long journey of my academic pursuit.

I am grateful to Mr. Stephen Leung, Mr. Chung Kin Man, Mr. Yuen Ming Ki, and Ms. Lau Mei Yan who helped in data collection, to Ms. Eva Kan who helped to do the test reliability and to Dr. Kong Luk, Dr. Y. H. Choy and Ms. Sue Yeung for proofreading the manuscript. I am also deeply indebted to my wife Nancy who supports me by sharing my responsibility at home. Finally, I must give my wholehearted thanks to God who provides me the opportunity to study and the perseverance to complete writing this book.

Andrew Leung LUK RN PhD
Director of Nethersole Institute of Continuing Holistic Health Education
Alice Ho Miu Ling Nethersole Charity Foundation

About the Author

Dr. LUK graduated from Queen Mary Hospital as a general nurse and obtained his post graduate training at Kwai Chung Hospital to be a psychiatric nurse. Being one of the founders of the Christian Oi Hip Fellowship in Hong Kong that provides holistic rehabilitation care to the ex-mental patients, he worked as a volunteer group counselor in the Fellowship for more than 16 years. His doctoral thesis was to evaluate the changes of the ex-mental patients attending the psychiatric rehabilitation program with holistic care and was found to be positive.

Dr. LUK has a strong commitment to the use of holistic principles in nursing. He has previously worked as a nursing administrator in Hong Kong and a nursing professor in Macau. He currently works as the director of Nethersole Institute of Continuing Holistic Health Education to promote holistic care in the Nethersole group of hospitals in Hong Kong.

PREFACE

It is well documented that persons with serious mental illness suffer from severe psychosocial issues. Besides these, studies suggest that many of them have different spiritual problems such as lacking of hope and losing meaning and purpose of life. In Hong Kong, a Christian non-governmental organization has developed a holistic care program for the rehabilitation of persons with serious mental illness. Holistic care is conceived as the care delivered to meet an integral, independent individual's health needs including physical, psychosocial, spiritual, cultural and environmental aspects as a whole. The holistic care program is characterized by a Self Help Group (SHG) approach with the adoption of holistic care principles where the physical, psychological, social and spiritual needs of the clients are emphasized. Beyond using solely conventional therapeutic intervention such as psychodynamic, cognitive and behavioural strategies in running SHGs, spiritual intervention in the form of hymn singing, Bible reading, personal sharing and intercessions is also used.

The holistic care rehabilitation program seeks to integrate Christian beliefs into every aspect of one's life through regularly scheduled meetings for mutual support. It is a partnership mode with mental health professionals as group leaders and persons with serious mental illness as members in running the group. All members are willing to share their problems and join the SHG voluntarily irrespective of their religious background. Each group member agrees to respect one and other's beliefs and not to impose his/her beliefs on another. Volunteer group leaders are mostly professionals including psychiatric nurses, social workers and occupational therapists, but some are non-professionals, who are recruited and specially trained by the organization to assist as co-leaders in the group. Established in 1990, the organization has formed 13 SHGs with more than 200 members actively participating in these groups.

Several studies have been conducted to measure the effectiveness of this holistic care program and showed that it is effective to provide some positive changes to its participants. A partnership model in SHG seems to be successful in providing support for the rehabilitation of persons with serious mental illness. Spiritual element should be incorporated into psychiatric rehabilitation program for instilling hope and meaningfulness of life. As spiritual care is an important component for persons with serious mental illness that may be neglected, spiritual beliefs should be included in mental health assessment and mental health professionals should be better educated in providing holistic care both to individual clients and to a group.

This book provides the theoretical background of the holistic care program, its format and development, and studies relating to measuring the effectiveness of the program. It can be used as a guidebook for the development of a holistic care program for those healthcare organizations which would like to offer long term support to persons with serious mental illness in the community.

Chapter 1

Background of the Development of a Holistic Care Program

It is well documented that individuals with serious mental illness suffer from severe psychosocial issues. The primary issue is directly due to psychiatric symptoms such as persistent hallucination and delusion; this is in addition to the adverse psychological reactions, such as low self-esteem and helplessness in response to one's illness. The secondary issue is caused by the stigmatization attached to being individuals with persistent and serious mental illness, which makes them difficult to integrate into the community (Stuart & Laraia, 2005, P. 242; Mezzina et al., 2006). Besides psychosocial issues, some local and overseas studies suggest, many individuals with serious mental illness have different spiritual problems, such as lacking hope (Landeen et al., 2000) and loss of the meaning and purpose of life (Lee et al., 1993; Leung, 1994; Kehoe, 2007). For example, in their proposed framework on spiritual assessment, Anandarajah and Hight (2001) suggested that hope and life meaning and their sources should be assessed.

With specific reference to Hong Kong, a review of the psychiatric rehabilitation system (Yip, 1996, 1997; Mak & Yip, 1997) shows a lacking of structured rehabilitation programs, especially the informal community programs based on the "self-help group" approach (SHG). Empirical research of SHGs in health related groups is limited. However, most local and overseas studies have shown them to be remarkably effective in promoting the recovery and rehabilitation of individuals who share common problems (Ma, 1992; Humphreys & Noke, 1997; Wituk et al., 2000; Mok, 2001; Clay, 2005). Furthermore, with the exception of the gospel drug rehabilitation programs (e.g., Ng & Shek, 2001), the spiritual element is not consciously included in most of the psychiatric rehabilitation programs.

In response to the above-mentioned deficiencies, there are some isolated services in Hong Kong that attempt to provide holistic psychiatric rehabilitation services to people with serious mental illness. One of the service providers is the Christian Oi Hip Fellowship (Fellowship), which is a Christian non-governmental organization providing holistic care programs for individuals with serious mental illness. The program is characterized by an SHG approach with the adoption of holistic care principles in which the physical, psychological, social, and spiritual needs of the clients are emphasized. This is where holistic care is conceived, as the care delivered meets the integral independent individual's health needs. This includes the physical, psychosocial, spiritual, cultural and environmental aspects of the individual patient as a whole (Hospital Authority 2001). Beyond using solely conventional therapeutic interventions such as psychodynamic, cognitive, and behavioral strategies in running SHGs, spiritual interventions in the form of hymn singing, Bible reading, personal sharing, and intercessions are also used.

The holistic care rehabilitation program in the Fellowship seeks to integrate Christian beliefs into every aspect of one's life through regularly scheduled meetings for mutual support. It is in the mode of a partnership consisting of mental health professionals as group leaders, along with individuals suffering from serious mental illness as members, collectively running the group. All members are willing to share their problems and join the SHG voluntarily irrespective of their religious background. Each group member agrees to respect one another's beliefs and not to impose his/her beliefs on another. Volunteer group leaders are mostly professionals including psychiatric nurses, social workers, and occupational therapists, but some are non-professionals, who are recruited and specially trained by the organization to assist as co-leaders in the group. They also agree to follow the rules of the Fellowship and to respect the faith of each member, regardless if the individual member, or the group, agrees with their Christian values and beliefs. Established in 1990, the Fellowship has formed 12 SHGs with more than 120 members actively participating in these groups. In 2008, there were 14 SHGs with more than 200 active members. Since the Fellowship has been developing for nearly 20 years, most of the groups are independent. They maintain their own activities through the group committee members without much involvement of the group leaders.

Chapter 2

HOLISTIC CARE IN HEALTHCARE PROFESSIONALS

2.1. DEFINITION OF HOLISTIC CARE

Towards the beginning of the new millennium, holistic care, which was once a heated topic discussed overseas during the end of the twentieth century, has become a topic of interest among the healthcare professionals in Hong Kong. In relation to medical treatment, Chinese medicine, a kind of holistic medicine, has been legitimatized in the health care system after the return of the sovereignty from the British government to the People Republic of China in 1997. In an era of the provision of high quality health services, holistic care for clients is an expectation of both the public and the healthcare professionals. However, the meaning of holistic care is subject to different interpretations especially in the dimension of spirituality.

In Christian beliefs, a man is viewed as a whole person consisting of three different parts of his own being: the spirit (Hebrew "ruah", Greek "pneuma"), the soul (Hebrew "nepes", Greek "psyche"), and the body (only in the New Testament Greek "soma"). However, they must not be regarded as separate or separable parts that make up what man is (Douglas et al., 1984, p. 731). The spirit is referred to as the immaterial part of man whereby a relationship with God is possible (Douglas et al., 1984, p. 1137). The soul refers to the immaterial part of man concerning the emotion, will, and moral action (Douglas et al., 1984, p. 1135). Lastly, the body denotes the principal constituent of the body, human, or animal (Douglas et al., 1984, pp. 145, 379). With a strong Christian heritage in western countries, the nature of man is always conceived of having the body, mind, and spirit. Hence, one of the common definitions of holism adopted by medical professionals, especially those with a Christian background, is a condition in which the human body, mind, and spirit are united in accomplishing health and well-being for the individual (Thompson, 1984).

Though there are different definitions of holistic care, the key component of a whole person including the body, mind, and spirit is always present in these definitions. As defined by some overseas nursing scholars, holistic care is care concerning a client's physical, psycho-social, and spiritual needs. The ultimate purpose of all health interventions is to enhance the quality of life that leads to the satisfaction of a client's external conditions of life and subjective experience to life (Lukkarinen & Hentinen, 1997). In Hong Kong, the Hospital Authority and some of its institutions have also developed their own definitions. Holistic care is defined as the care delivered to meet an integral, independent individual's health needs including physical, psycho-social, spiritual, cultural, and environmental aspects as a whole (Hospital Authority, 2001). Holistic care is a philosophy and practice of compassionate care, which respects the value and dignity of man and upholds the physical, psychological, social, and spiritual well-being of the total person (AHNH, 2001).

The definition provided by the Hospital Authority is adopted in this book, since they are the largest healthcare provider in Hong Kong, providing for more than 90% of the healthcare services. The appreciation of a patient as biological, psychological, and social, as well as a spiritual being is one of the major characteristics of holistic medicine (Gordon 1980). As argued by Gordon (1990), the concept of holism is a powerful one, appealing to lay people who feel their health care is fragmented and to health care professionals who crave for a more integrated and individual practice. Holistic medicine attempts to include all the techniques that modern science and empirical use have found to be helpful. However, those treatment modalities that do not come from conventional (orthodox or allopathic) western scientific medicine are termed under "complementary or alternative medicines" (CAM) (Forbes, 2000). These include some which are more scientific based such as biofeedback (Renshaw, 1984), meditation, psychotherapy, behavior modification, ancient acupuncture, massage (Aston, 1984), and visualization (Pownal, 1986). Others such as prayer, reflexology, tai chi, yoga, aroma-therapy, and herbal medicine, which are under studied or without sound scientific bases, are also commonly used. A study conducted by Eisenberg et al., (1998) showed that the number of Americans who reported using CAM as part of their health regimen increased to nearly 47%. Bowler (2008) reported that there was an exponential growth and popularity of CAM in the U.K. with an estimated 19 million people using it, which sits firmly within the mainstream of healthcare provision in the U.K.

2.2. THE RISE OF HOLISTIC MEDICINE

Primitive humans sought both natural and supernatural means to treat illness. Primitive medicines made from vegetables or animals were invariably used in combination with some form of ritual to expel the harmful spirit from a diseased body. Therefore, suggested by DuBos (1969), medicine has had a dual nature from its inception. It included knowledge-based practice and a belief in some magic or religious power involving forces beyond human comprehension. It is also stated by Guthrie (1945), one of the leading medical historians, that medicine was first in the hands of the priest. It was not until around 400 B.C., that the Greek physician Hippocrates formulated the principles and practices of medicine based upon rational thought and rejected the supernatural phenomena. During the Middle Ages and Renaissance, the mind became the domain of study by the Church, while the role of the physician was to focus exclusively on treating problems of the human body (Cockerham, 1986). The lack of understanding of psychological and social factors in illnesses continued during the seventeenth century. In the 1800s, the discovery of the germ theory, along with the rapid development of medical science, reinforced physicians to concentrate on improving the state of medical technology. In the 1940s, the introduction of antibiotics and tranquilizers revolutionized the pharmacological approach, which is still dominant nowadays in Western medicine. At the same time, technology was also improved both to anaesthetize patients and to perform very complex operative procedures (Shealy, 2000). The practice of medicine in the twentieth century thus rested solidly upon a biomedical framework.

Holism was first coined by Smuts (1926) in his book, from which holistic medicine derives its name. To Smuts, holism is a way of comprehending the whole organism and biological systems as entities greater than and different from the sum of their parts, which was an antidote to the reductionism of contemporary science. Dubos (1959), a microbiologist, first articulated that modern medicine had far less to do with improving our health than did changes in nutrition, sanitation, and life-style. Illich (1977), a theologian, provided substantial lists of the 'harmful side effects' of many drugs, and of 'unnecessary surgery'. He argued that chemotherapy and surgery were actually new forms of an epidemic and that scientific medicine had made all of us patients.

Furthermore, during the middle of the twentieth century, the area of the psychosomatic medicine had demonstrated the power of mind over matter and *vice versa*. It is clear that mind and body are so closely interconnected that it is no longer appropriate to view illness merely as a state of the body. It is the whole person who falls ill, not a body or some body system or an organ. Thus, there is recognition of the "bio-psychosocial" approach to health care (Engel, 1977). Health is then defined as a complete physical, mental, and social well-being and not merely the absence of disease and infirmity (W.H.O. 1947).

As medicine moves toward the twenty-first century, a new definition of man including a fourth dimension is emerging, the spiritual. This enlarges the bio-psychosocial domain and redefines the nature and purpose of treatment and care for patients. As suggested by Relman (1979), the most startling manifesto of the holistic movement is a published volume entitled, "Wholistic Dimensions in Healing" (Kaslof, 1978). It purports to be a "resource guide", briefly explaining the various "alternative" approaches to health care and listing related groups and publications that can be consulted by the public for further help and information. Aldridge (1993), as a research psychologist, argued that many clinical cases with issues of abandonment, suffering, loss of hope and meaning, and the transition from living to dying are essentially spiritual, and clearly not solely physiological, psychological, or social. In a national survey by Bergin & Jensen (1990) with samples including psychologists, psychiatrists, social workers, and marriage and family therapists, 29% agreed that religious issues are important in the treatment of all or many of their clients. Anderson and Young (1988) claimed that, "all clinicians inevitably face the challenge of treating patients with religious troubles and preoccupation" (p. 532). Observations made by nursing colleagues ascertained that diseases, no matter acute or chronic, resulted in a loss of identity, self-control, acceptance, and often meaning of life, caused a disharmony of body, mind, and spirit (Collitan, 1981).

As suggested by Fuller (1996), the holistic healing movement throughout the 1970s is "rife with symbols evoking an explicitly spiritual interpretation of the healing process" (p. 239). The basic premise of the holistic approach to healing is relatively straightforward and it appears to be little more than another means of expressing Americans eager to re-humanize their technological society: "Every human being is a unique, holistic, interdependent relationship of body, mind, emotions, and spirit" (Belknap et al., 1975, p. 18).

Gordon (1982) offered seven characteristics of holistic medicine:

1. Each patient is treated as a unique individual made up of body, mind, and spirit, and provision of health care must also take into account a person's environment.
2. It emphasizes each person's responsibility to his/her health.
3. It includes the promotion of health, the prevention of disease and health education.
4. A variety of treatment modalities that lies outside the conventional western medical practice is also used.
5. It emphasizes the contribution of therapeutic environment.
6. It stresses the importance of those social and economic conditions that perpetuate ill health.
7. It is concerned with educating physicians to broaden and enrich their medical practice.

On the one hand, holistic medicine emphasizes the psychological factors that promote regeneration and well-being. It is suggested that the patient generally has difficulty coping with the condition and is in desperate need of love, care, and understanding. It is therefore essential for health care providers to give "abundantly of their warmth, empathy and understanding and furnish the type of emotional nurturance particularly needed at a time of illness" (Otto & Knight, 1979, p. 3). On the other hand, the introduction of the term spirit alongside body, mind, and emotions takes the holistic conceptions of healing well beyond the psychosomatic models and marks a bold metaphysical interpretation of reality. The acceptance of the relationship and influence between the physical and non-physical spheres makes holistic not only an alternative approach to medicine but an alternative way to view the world.

Otto and Knight (1979) described holistic medicine as advocating that every human being had vast untapped potential, resources, and powers which were not self-contained within the physical or psychological system. Rather, "everyone is part of a larger system." Holistic healing must utilize the patient's spiritual resources to help "to open the pathways or flows and harmonics necessary to unfold the channels of the self within the body and the self within the world, the Universe, and God" (Otto & Knight, 1979, p. 10). Thus, proponents of holistic medicine not only acknowledge the body's self-recuperative abilities, but also gradually accept that the body is receptive to the healing energies flowing into it from without.

Of course, not every practice of alternative medicine propounds a spiritual mode of healing. However, the fact remains that most practices consist of this alternative world view. To quote a few examples: The Chiropractors by Palmer (1910), The Therapeutic Touch by Krieger (1979) and the Alcoholic Anonymous by Bill W. (Alcoholics Anonymous, 1955). Alcoholics Anonymous (AA) is the most illustrative example of holistic medicine. Participants are guided to acquire "an overwhelming 'God-consciousness' followed at once by a vast change in feeling and outlook" (Alcoholics Anonymous, 1955, p. 569). Alcoholic Anonymous warns against the attempt to rely on self-sufficiency. It maintains that the key to personal regeneration is attainment of the "feeling of being at one with God and man" (Twelve Steps and Twelve Traditions, 1952, p. 63). As stated by Fuller (1996), the founder of AA, Bill W., was wary of organized religion, knowing that many alcoholics are painfully conscious of their inability to live up to the moral absolutes associated with biblical religion. Instead, he sought to articulate a spiritual approach to personal regeneration that was free of dogmas and fixed traditions. The "Twelve Step" program is a unique blend of mysticism and pragmatism pieced together from the writings of such religiously oriented psychologists as William James and Carl Jung. Referring to itself as "spiritual rather than religious," AA is a prime carrier of America's secular spiritual heritage that stresses true self-reliance is possible only once we have experientially connected ourselves with the Other: "The more we become willing to depend upon a higher power, the more independent we actually are" (Twelve Steps and Twelve Traditions, 1952, p. 7). The AA non-biblical approach to spiritual regeneration arouses criticism from most of America's religious establishments. Furthermore, it is the denial of the usefulness of physical and psychological treatment, instead of the metaphysical means for healing that also leads to attacks from American medical establishments. However, the open-minded and eclectic approach of using spiritual forces for human well-being makes it one of the most powerful mediators of wholeness in America (Fuller, 1996).

In short, Fergusson (1995) suggested several reasons for the rise of holistic medicine: 1) failure of orthodox medicine to offer a cure of diseases especially of chronic illnesses and cancer; 2) the arrogance of many western medical practitioners in ignoring failure, and refusing to come to terms with the limitations of medical treatment; 3) the commonness of iatrogenic disease due to the presence of side effects with the increasing powerful treatments, while most of the alternative medicines are physically harmless; 4) the loss of the holistic approach is seen specifically in shortness of time, lack of touch and trust; and finally 5) most alternative medicines are rather cheap, but mainly requiring the therapist's time.

In Hong Kong, upon the return of sovereignty from Britain to China, the Hong Kong Special Administration Region endeavors to promote Traditional Chinese Medicine (TCM) that is originated from the ancient Chinese yin/yang philosophy. With its historical roots in Taoism and Buddhism, TCM stresses on the wholeness of body, mind, and spirit, and the unity of the individual with the natural environment. It asserts that all physiological processes are governed by spiritual agency that emanates from the divine (Tao) (Pelletier, 1973). The central concept of Chinese medicine is Qi, which is the vital energy, or life force that animates all living beings and the entire universe. The underlying belief of TCM is that Qi travels through a system of energy channels, or meridians, which flow along the surface of the body and through the internal organs. If any of these meridians is blocked, pain or other disease can occur. TCM also emphasizes the importance of the polarity of yin and yang entities. Yin is associated with the feminine, passive, dark, and inner qualities. Yang is related to the masculine, active, light, and outer qualities. In order to be healthy, one must have a balance between yin and yang. Acupuncture, as one modality of TCM, is used to balance yin and yang by influencing the flow of Qi energy through the body (Pelletier, 2000).

2.3. Criticisms of the Concept of Holistic Medicine

During the evolution of holistic medicine, it has come under attack on a number of grounds by some physicians. Relman (1979) warned that there was an irrational side of the holistic movement, with its mystical cults and as a collection of obscure and unproved modalities and ancient truisms. Though there is no argument concerning treating a person as a whole person, this worthwhile philosophy is ill-served by those who seek quick solutions to all the ills of mankind through the abandonment of science and rationality in favor of mystical cults. Additionally, it should be cautioned not to turn medicine "From Science to Sects" in the history of the holistic movement. Callan (1979) argued that holistic medicine advocated "complete wellness" which was difficult to demonstrate by objective scientific means. Besides, the goal of complete personal fulfillment seemed to be unrealistic or grandiose. Furthermore, many holistic practitioners had a polished rhetoric and supported arguments from medical authorities with their own superlatives. Physicians should take precautions about its development.

In the same vein, Yahn (1979), a physician in private practice, commented that some physicians formed holistic medical centers or clinics sometimes inviting non-physician healthcare professionals to join. Some of these non-physicians were not licensed, and no standards were set up. It has been recommended that immediate steps should be taken to regulate holistic practitioners by licensing to eliminate those who are improperly qualified. Standards should also be devised to determine whether these non-physician holistic practitioners are practicing legitimate healthcare. It was further commented that there were also commercialistic tendencies and faddism in some centers. Some literature from these centers had been criticized as unscientific and being written for laymen by laymen. Crawford (1977) argued that the rise of holistic care was due to the emergence of the new victim blaming ideology that blamed the individual for her or his illness. He proposed that, instead of relying on costly and inefficient medical services, the individual should take more responsibility for her or his health and it would be unwise to over-emphasize the abandonment of medicine. Although physicians are a primary source of such criticism, holistic medicine has become more popular and its advocates more vocal.

Most negative arguments of holistic medicine focus on the unscientific base of its treatment modality, as compared with western medicine that is mainly evidence based. In fact, not all treatment in western medicine is scientifically sound, and evidence-based medicine is very much emphasized in advanced medical practice. Furthermore, some types of holistic medicine such as acupuncture, therapeutic touch, tai chi, etc. have been studied and shown to be effective in maintaining health. At present, many medical schools have set up centers of Complementary and Alternative Medicine for scientific studies. In the foreseeable future, more treatment modalities of holistic medicine will also be evidence based. Another argument is on the control of holistic medical practice that is not performed by physician. It is reasonable that only qualified personnel with an acceptable standard should carry out all medical practice. But the main point is that customers have their choices. It is the inadequacy of western medicine that causes the customers to seek help from an alternative therapist. It would be the responsibilities of the physicians to develop a trusting relationship with their patients and render an effective service. However, as advocated by Ernst (2006), we should be cautious about the potential of alternative treatment in boosting pseudoscience and be alert about the scientific bases of those positive studies.

To sum up, most practices of alternative medicine are concerned with the healing of the whole person and awakening the spirit within. Despite their differences, each utilizes techniques with the belief that humans are all affected by the universal life energy. Holistic or alternative medicine is not simply referring to a different set of material factors dismissed as unimportant by the medical establishment. Instead, they are concerned with pushing any conception of healing to the point that discloses the ultimate meaning or significance of our lives. In other words, the holistic view acknowledges objective, scientific explanations of physiology, but 'also acknowledges that people have inner experiences that are subjective, mystical and for some religious…. which may affect health' (Edlin & Golanty, 1992). This holistic view not only arises in medicine, but also extends its influence in different healthcare disciplines. Nevertheless, the main argument is still whether the practice is scientifically sound or not. Since evidence-based practice is indispensable, in this book it is important to look at the changes that have occurred in the participants of the holistic care program offered by the Fellowship.

2.4. Holistic Care in Nursing and Social Work: Current Status And Implications

Nursing

The concept of holistic care is not a new phenomenon in nursing. Many authors underline the longstanding tradition of a holistic philosophy in nursing (Allen, 1991a, 1991b; Lynaugh & Fagin, 1988; Martin, 1986; McGuire, 1990). Although the term "holism" was not yet used, holistic notions were already applied to conceptualize the role of the nurse at the turn of the century, especially in public health nursing (Allen, 1991a, 1991b; Wald, 1915). The word holism was first used by Smuts (1926), a South African scientist, who reflected on the states of that country, and concluded that they were greater as South Africa than as separate states (Owen & Holmes, 1993). Though there is no succinct definition, the most generally accepted understanding is that the 'whole is greater than the sum of its parts'.

As illustrated by Barnum (1995), nursing has an interesting history in which it intertwines itself with spirituality and can trace its origins to the spirituality arising from ancient religions. However, the religious origins of nursing were lost due to systematic sacrifices in the name of professionalism and the scientific worldview. During 1970s, the holistic health movement attracted health practitioners who were dissatisfied with the objectifying aspects of the dominant biomedical approach. They associated the biomedical model with reductionistic, atomistic, dualistic, and mechanistic thought, and an authoritarian approach to patients (Blattner, 1981; Lowenberg, 1989).

Holistic nursing is advocated as a key philosophy in promoting disease prevention and health-seeking behaviors. Johnson (1990) described the diffusion of holistic ideas into nursing practice during the last two decades. According to her analysis, various aspects of holistic nursing can be identified: the integration, harmony, and balance of body, mind, and spirit; a focus on wholeness of the individual with emphasis on the process of self-healing rather than on disease; illness as an opportunity for growth and increased self-awareness; and the reciprocal relationship between nurse and patient with emphasis on self-responsibility, health promotion, and lifestyle (Johnson, 1990). Sarkis and Skloner (1987) and Johnson (1990), found that in recent decades more concepts from alternative healing practices were included in the holistic perspective of nursing.

The American Holistic Nursing Association (AHNA) was founded in 1981 to promote the education of nurses, other healthcare professionals, and the public in all aspects of holistic care and healing. The Journal of Holistic Nursing, a peer-reviewed journal, was also established in 1983 to provide a platform for nurses to exchange information, share experiences, and communicate research relating to holistic nursing practices and health care. It has been a pioneering force in integrating holistic health concepts with traditional Western medicine. At present, the AHNA has over 5,700 members in U.S. (AHNA, 2012).

Social Work

Viewing from the historical roots of the social work profession, the early stages of social work were solidly embedded in the rich Judeo-Christian heritage (Leiby, 1985). Many religious organizations worked to establish orphanages, hospitals, schools, and numerous other services. Likewise, many social work professionals had religious backgrounds. Holland (1989) maintained that most of the original social work practitioners were spiritually motivated and committed to express their faith through their services to the needy. Ortiz (1991) argued that many fundamental values of the profession such as love and justice came out of the Judeo-Christian tradition, and Canda (1988a) also supported that social work practice had its roots in religious activities.

With strong Christian heritage, the concept of holism is also embedded in the practice of social work. Even though the social work profession has made conscious attempts to avoid addressing religious or spiritual issues, owing to the emphasis on the scientific objective practice in the 18th and 19th centuries (Graham et al., 1998). Towle (1965) suggested that common human needs were those needs that were shared by all human beings because they were basic to their survival and development. They included physical well-being, personality development, emotional growth, development of intellectual capacity, relationships with others, and spiritual needs. The spiritual needs of the individual must also be recognized, understood, and respected. Through the influence of religion, the purpose of human life is better understood and a sense of ethical value is achieved (pp. 6-11). Bardill (1976) maintained that the human consists of four interconnected domains and functional human behavior is derived from the realistic consideration of all four relational areas. The four domains were: 1) self, which is defined as subjective reality, 2) other, which is defined as the world of physical objects and states, both organic and inorganic, 3) context, which is defined as the world in the objective sense, and 4) spiritual, which is defined as the supreme force that governs the universe.

There have been increasing influences of holistic medicine to healthcare and social work professionals. Most of them are extending their roles to render holistic care to their clients (Coulon et al., 1996; Graham et al., 1998; Hawley & Irurita, 1998; Kilpatrick & Holland, 1990; Hemphill-Pearson & Hunter, 1997; Ross, 1997). However, in practice, the concept towards holistic care varies especially in the spiritual perspective. Many authors in varied fields such as nursing, social work, sociology, psychology, theology, physics, and philosophy have attempted to conceptualize and operationalize the spiritual dimension, but actual definitions vary since the concept of spirituality is hard to grasp (Canda, 1988b; Carson, 1989; Fischer, 1985; Frankl, 1963; Hiatt, 1986; Joseph, 1987; Moberg, 1979). In the following section, conceptions of spirituality in social science theories will be examined, and the spiritual dimension of the whole person will be explored in relation to helping professionals and the treatment of clients, particularly in the context of nursing and social work.

Chapter 3

Conceptions of Spirituality in Social Science Theories

Different views on spirituality have been expressed by different social scientists and studies are carried out for supporting different arguments. In the following discussion, spirituality in some major perspective of psychology and sociology will be examined.

3.1. Psychological Theories

William James (1961), being the most prominent psychologist in the psychological study of religion, contributes to our understanding of the relationship of religion and spirituality. He defined religion as "the feelings, acts, and experiences of individual men in their solitude, so far as they apprehend themselves to stand in relation to whatever they may consider the divine" (p. 42). Within this framework, James analyzed the various ways that personal "religious life," although subject to considerable distortion and perversity, represented a set of belief experiences linking individual humans to "a more spiritual universe" from which they drew significance. Understood in this way, religious life, James concluded, enriched the believer through prayer, which was a source of "spiritual energy…a zest which added itself like a gift to life, a temper of peace, and loving affections toward others" (p. 377). Furthermore, he viewed that religion could alleviate human suffering by providing understanding and solutions to the problem of human misery and fallibility, the factor which might maintain the existence of religion in society.

Transpersonal perspective

In modern psychology, it is found that the spiritual dimension of man is an area worth exploring and a branch of transpersonal psychology is being developed. It applies scientific methods to those areas of human experience beyond the strictly empirical, such as mystical experience, transcendence of self, spirit and spiritual practices, meditation, and compassion based in a cosmic consciousness. Transpersonal psychology is concerned with developing a self, while also honoring the urge to go beyond the self (Cortright, 1997, p. 9). Strohl (1998) cites Lajoie and Shapiro's definition of transpersonal psychology as being "concerned with the study of humanity's highest potential, and with the recognition, understanding, and realization of unitive, spiritual, and transcendent states of consciousness" (p. 397).

Transpersonal psychology has its origins in the 1960s in the United States. Emerging from humanistic and existential psychology, transpersonal psychology, currently encompasses the wisdom of the world religions toward the expansion of human consciousness and fulfillment of human potentialities (Cortright, 1997). It is also suggested to be the "fourth force" in psychology, building upon the psychoanalytic, behavioral, and humanistic movements. As Maslow and others continued humanistic research and therapy, they found that many people who showed high levels of life satisfaction also reported important transformative events that moved them to explicit spiritual interests (Canda & Furman, 1999). Robbins et al., (1998) put it, "They discovered that many highly self-actualized people reported experiences of self-transcendence that were, paradoxically, crucial to their sense for self-fulfillment. These experiences are termed transpersonal because they transcend the limits of the 'persona,' ego-bounded self-identity" (p. 360).

Transpersonal theory focuses on understanding the altered states of consciousness, the spiritual development process, and therapeutic techniques that facilitate transpersonal awareness. Transpersonalists suggest that the transpersonal self recognizes that true self-actualization is inseparable from other-actualization. Depending on the spiritual perspective of the person, the ultimate level of development may be described as a union with God, unity of true self with the true nature of the universe, enlightenment, or cosmic consciousness. Some transpersonalists view all these descriptions as different religious or philosophical terminology for the same mystical experience (Canda & Furman, 1999).

Some prominent psychologists in this area, as highlighted by Kelly (1995), are as follows: Assagioli (1971, 1993) started his seminal work in psycho-synthesis and developed an influential transpersonal model for the integration of spirituality and psychotherapy. Having earlier experiences with psychedelic drugs, Grof and Grof (1989) developed transpersonal counseling applications that explored theoretical and clinical distinctions between beneficially transformative spiritual experiences and pseudo-spiritual experiences rooted in mental disorders. Wilber et al., (1986) worked on the eastern religious experience and eastern psychology and also had integrated eastern thought with western psychology.

Though some psychologists hold a positive view towards spirituality, many are on the negative side. They postulate that all problems are basically psychological or even physical, in another term, the dichotomistic view of persons. Psychological reductionism maintains that through spirituality, in a narrow sense, religion has provided a pre-scientific perspective on individuals that is more fully and accurately presented in modern psychology. The major perspectives of psychology discussed below include psychoanalytic, behavioral, cognitive, and existential views.

Psychoanalytic perspective

Freud

Freud, the founder of psychoanalysis, viewed spirits and demons as "projections of man's non-emotional impulses" (1913, p. 92) and God as the "displacement of oedipal ambivalence and as a cosmic projection of the father complex" (1910, p. 123). He also saw religion as "a system of wishful illusions together with a disavowal of reality, such as we find…nowhere else…but a state of blissful hallucinatory confusion" and a "universal obsessional neurosis" (Freud, 1966). Freud viewed religion as an illusion. God is a projection of humans' infantile wishes rooted in the father-complex; religion is an obsessional neurosis with neurotic wishes expressed in ritualistic compulsions. That religion is contrary to human progress, and the moral aspects of religion should be replaced with science and non-theistic humanism.

Wallace (1983) criticized that Freud's "psycho-pathologizing" of religion reflects his personal judgments, which were not based on the results of his psychoanalytic work with religious patients but were a speculative extrapolation of his own ideas, prejudices, and religious conflicts. Moreover, Wallace pointed out that while Freud might have been correct in noting some similarities between religion and neurosis, he failed to correctly understand the significance of this similarity. Critiques from modern anthropological investigations and historical evidence pointed clearly to a non-conclusive link between Freud's major psychoanalytical principles and his explanations of religion (Kung, 1981). However, his critique of religion had positive aspects that were important to the understanding of potentially negative and detrimental effects of religion. These effects were summarized by Kung (1979) as follows: 1) the defective forms of religion and their psychological effects including self-deception, escapism, satisfaction of personal needs through wish fulfillment, religious legalism and ritualism that narrowed one's range of thinking and behaving. 2) Institutional religion's misuse of power and influence. 3) Domination or intimidation of the human spirit in the name of God and the exploitation of those who are dependent, immature, psychologically or spiritually vulnerable.

Fromm

Fromm (1950), a Neo-Freudian and one of the prominent humanistic psychologists, argued psychology was better able to explain and solve the problems and phenomena encountered by religion. He stated, "The psychoanalyst is in a position to study the human reality behind religion as well as behind non-religious symbol systems. He finds that the question is not whether man returns to religion and believes in God but whether he lives love and thinks truth. If he does so the symbol systems he uses are of secondary importance. If he does not they are of no importance" (Fromm, 1950, p. 9). Fromm thus viewed religion with tolerance but also with condescension, inferring that psychotherapy would accomplish the same ends as religion, but it did so without the trappings of dogma or religious symbols.

Fromm (1950) proposed that "humanistic" religion had human self-realization and growth in one's specifically human powers of reason and love as its aim and was therefore productive and progressive. "Authoritarian" religion, on the other hand, was based on irrational submissiveness to authority; it thus alienated the individual from himself since he projects all his own productive powers onto God and is therefore non-productive and regressive. For Fromm, the ultimate criterion for evaluating religious faith was not the objective validity of the content of one's faith but the human experience of the believer. It is a question of whether one's faith expresses itself in productive or non-productive living; whether it helps the believer to become more fully human or to retreat from his humanity. For humanistic religion virtue is defined as "self-realization, not obedience," faith is not "certainty of conviction" but a certainty based on one's own experience and thought, not on submissiveness to a teaching authority; God is "a symbol of man's own powers which he tries to realize in his life, and is not a symbol of force and domination having power over man" (Fromm, 1950, p. 37). Thus, Fromm is equally critical of what he perceives as the emphasis on human powerlessness in the Lutheran and Calvinist traditions and of the emphasis on an infallible teaching authority in the Catholic tradition. These are viewed as a craving for certainty at the expense of independence and personal responsibility to one's life.

However, argued by Forsyth (1997), Fromm "fails to differentiate between religion and religious experience. Religious experience may be judged to be either humanistic or authoritarian since the believer may assimilate his religious tradition in a way that is psychologically healthy or unhealthy. But for precisely the same reason it is difficult to apply the same criterion to a religious tradition as such" (p. 181).

Jung

The Neo-Freudian, on the other hand, viewed spirituality in a more positive way. Jung (1936) argued that both analysis and pastoral care were concerned with the cure of souls. However, he went on to distinguish between them by suggesting that while analysis cures souls by reinforcing the natural drive toward wholeness that exists within a person, pastoral care, in other words, religion, supplies answers and meaning that are outside the individual.

Jung demonstrated that spirituality is rooted in personality and thereby provides a preliminary map of the relationship between spirituality and psychology. The central concept in Jung's view of spirituality as illustrated by Benner (1988) is that of individuation – the life-long process of becoming whole through the synthesis of conscious and unconscious aspects of personality. The ego is the center of the consciousness, while the self is the innermost center of the unconscious extending beyond consciousness. Jung postulated that both spiritual and psychological health depends on an open relationship between the conscious and unconscious forces in personality. However, the conscious part of the personality is only a way station toward integration but people tend to get stuck in ego-centeredness and wholeness that is the goal of the spiritual quest, which can only be obtained from movement to the self as center.

The divine, in accordance with Jung's view, is essentially an inner character of the mind, like everything else, occurs as an intra-psychic image. God is an intra-psychic force appearing to consciousness in symbolic form. Jung rejected the view that divine figures exist outside the psyche, which was the totality of all psychic processes. However, Jung also had quite a lot to say about conditions outside the psyche. Through the doctrine of the microcosmic character of the psyche, Jung identified individual human life with the universe as a whole. Fuller (1994) argued, "By defining the individual in cosmic terms, Jung leaves far behind the modest claims of an empiricist only interested in the phenomena. Jung's psychology turns out in fact to be pantheistic metaphysics" (p. 111).

Besides, Jung's conceptualization of spirituality is also criticized by many Christian psychologists to be away from the Christian beliefs. "Jung's is a religious doctrine in which God is rendered completely interior. The 'Thou' term becomes a function of the 'I' (Rieff, 1966, p. 97). In the progress of spiritual growth, self is deified and God is psychologized. According to Doran (1979), Jung interprets the innermost center not in terms of God's grace but of nature. While suggested by Kopas (1981, p. 220), Jung builds self-transcendence into his model, in actuality he remains much closer to self-fulfillment. Anyway, his focus is basically on natural spirituality, that is, the native soil out of which either genuine Christian spirituality or some alternate spirituality develops.

Behavioral perspective

Skinner

Skinnerian behaviorism ignores the religious experience to focus exclusively on observable behavior (Watson, 1930). In response to the religiously oriented Alcoholics Anonymous (AA) steps, Skinner (1977) seriously objected and wrote a "Twelve-Step Humanist" alternative program, which he sent to AA for their consideration. In Skinner's program, friend replaces the concept of a higher power or God, and self-control was once again re-emphasized. Skinner's own approach to behavioral research is characterized by concentration upon single subjects, automated equipment and well-defined control over experimental conditions. It is criticized as a narrowness view in understanding human behavior. Furthermore, to conceive of human actions solely in terms of stimulus input and response output may be adequate for the study of very simple forms of behavior, but this approach neglects too many interesting areas of human functioning (Hilgard et al., 1979). Bufford (1981), in his attempt to reconcile behavioral psychology with Christian theology, suggested that the simplest or most basic explanation did not make all high levels of analysis and their respective explanations redundant, but that they complemented each other. As suggested by Thyer and Hudson (1987), though behavior approaches have been applied in substantive problem areas by professional social workers, they "may or may not subscribe to the philosophy of behaviorism" (p. 1).

Cognitive perspective

Ellis

Albert Ellis, the originator of rational emotive (cognitive) therapy, also views religion as equivalent to irrational thinking and emotional disturbances. "The elegant therapeutic solution to emotional problems is quite unreligious....The less religious (clients) they are, the more emotionally healthy they will tend to be" (Ellis, 1980, p. 637). Ellis maintains that atheism, although not absolutely demonstrable, is nonetheless about 99% probable, thereby overwhelmingly representing a more rational, more truly human, basis for living one's life (Ellis, 1989). According to this perspective, belief in spiritual and religious entities is irrational and constitutes a psychological deficit for the individual, and in its institutional forms, an obstruction to social well-being.

Alcoholics Anonymous (AA) has helped millions of addicts since its founding in 1935. However, argued by Ellis and Schoenfeld (1990), it had turned away even more because of its emphasis on a higher power. Furthermore, there is real harm in retaining those steps dealing with the AA concept of God. In response to Step 2 of the Twelve Steps of AA, "came to believe that a power greater than ourselves could restore us to sanity", he argued that it was much more useful and universally applicable to instruct patients that there were outside powers who could help restore one to sanity, not necessarily a higher power, but others of different powers, for example, physicians or therapists. Relating to Step 6, "were entirely ready to have God remove all these defects of character", it was argued that this step reinforced dependency outside oneself, which was not a drug but God. Ellis opposed that AA's reliance on a supernatural higher power showed no confidence in the ability of addicts to abet their own growth and development and to help themselves.

However, Kelly (1995) argued both theism and atheism could be a choice of illusion. Since the atheistic position does not draw the conclusion from evidence, it could be "a choice to reject the theistic or spiritual implications of psychological experience and physical evidence pointing to an objective reality corresponding to ultimate transcendent meaning" (p. 56). For example, atheism could be a repression of trust and affirmation that the universe is really and ultimately meaningful. Relating to probabilities, Kelly further argued that the probabilities regarding theism and atheism are closer to 50-50, in contrast to Ellis's assertion.

Cited by Kelly (1995), there are many examples which show themselves as reasonable as the unbeliever's denial such as, "serious arguments made for an innate sense of the sacred ("drive to find God") in human knowledge (Liddon, 1989); the meta-empirical outreaches of scientific probing of the universe (Davies, 1992); the extensively positive compatibility of the spiritual /religious worldview with the subject matter and practice of psychology (Jones, 1994) and the believer's affirmation of ultimate transcendence (variously named God, the divine, spirituality, and other terms), all show themselves as reasonable as the unbeliever's denial" (p. 57). In a cognitive model of religion's influence on health described by Dull and Skokan (1995), it is suggested that religious beliefs may influence health through either of two processes: 1) by recommending specific prescriptions for health maintaining behaviors, and 2) by supporting cognition that affect stress appraisal and physiology. Then, the role of religious beliefs and cognition may serve a dual role in the efficacious or deleterious impact on health.

Existential perspective

Kierkegaard

The existentialist Kierkegaard views individuals as spirits. While "spirit" is the "self-relating to itself" (Kierkegaard, 1954, p. 146), self is referring to self-acceptance, self-understanding, and self-consciousness, all qualities of a growing self or spirit. But he postulates that self cannot become all it is intended to be by itself. Ultimately, self can only become a true self by relating itself to God (1954, p. 162). For Kierkegaard, self is a synthesis of all parts of personality, even those that are not easily put together. The struggle to bring these discrepant parts together is a spiritual struggle by which one becomes one true self, rather than living out the false self. He further states that, "consciousness of self is the criterion of self. The more consciousness, the more self"(1954, p. 162). However, he makes it explicit the way in which knowledge of God is a part of this process, "The more conception of God, the more self; the more self, the more conception of God. Only when the self as this definite individual is conscious of existing before God, only then is it the infinite self" (1954, p. 211).

Frankl

Another prominent existentialist, Viktor Frankl (1963), is famous for his psychotherapeutic technique, the logotherapy, which aims at the discovery of the concrete meaning of a person's existence. In doing so, he states that it, "dares to enter the spiritual dimension of human existence." It deals with the spiritual issues, namely, "man's aspirations for a meaningful existence, as well as the frustration of this aspiration." In fact, Frankl views human personality as a three-dimensional reality: the physical, the psychological, and the spiritual. The physical dimension refers to the operation of the physiological systems such as nervous system, the psychological to the instincts and drives and the spiritual to the striving for meaningful existence.

Forsyth (1997) highlights two main points of Frankl's understanding of human personality. Firstly, "will to meaning" is the most basic motivating force in human personality. It is the desire to live a meaningful existence and to discover the reasons of one's personal existence. The second is that the "spiritual dimension" of human personality is revealed beyond the physical and psychological (instinctive) dimensions. Thus, the search for meaning, a kind of conscious spiritual activity is not merely a sublimation of the instinctual unconscious but springs from the "spiritual unconscious". It is more fundamental to human existence than the instinctual will to pleasure. Self-transcendence takes place when one finds the meaning of his existence. Recently, the basic principles of logotherapy has been translated and extended into cognitive behavioral processes and a new form of logotherapy "meaning-centered" counseling has been developed in social work practice (Wong, 1998).

3.2. SOCIOLOGICAL THEORIES

Different sociologists also express different views towards spirituality or religion. From the function perspective of sociology, Karl Marx, the founder of Communism, views religion as "false consciousness," since it deals with what is either trivial or nonexistent and really reflects the economic interests of the dominant social class (Wood, 1981, pp. 12-15). Religion is seen as the "opiate of the people" because it offers them a "pie in the sky" to divert them from the class struggle and prolong their exploitation. However, another famous sociologist, Max Weber, challenges this view. Weber (1930) examined the rise of capitalism and argued that it was favored by the attitudes stressed by ascetic Protestantism. Thus, rather than religion being without real influence, it actually helped to formulate the direction of economic change. Weber (1922) viewed religion as a sort of institution with a socially shared set of cognition, which provided in turn a guide to life, a definition of self and a general interpretation of reality for the individual. Sharing with a positive view, Durkheim (1961) identified five basic functions of religion in society: 1) religion legitimizes social norms, 2) religion provides a sense of shared experience and solidarity for its members, 3) religion assists people in adjusting to life crises and hardships, 4) religious worship seals the bonds of solidarity between members of a society, 5) religion offers support in times of accelerated social change and disorganization. In a parallel view, Parsons (1960) stated that one of the major functions of religion in society was to regulate the individual's motivational commitment to social values, thus mediating the person's role in society.

Regarding social work practice, toward the development of a theory, the strengths perspective of social work, works on client strengths as a whole, including spirituality. By focusing work on client strengths such as talents, knowledge, capacities, resources, etc., in the assessment and planning process, problems are less likely to be invented or exacerbated. Through the collaborative process between the social worker and the client, the client not only manages to overcome his/her problems, but also can find meaning and experience a personal growth with hope and transformation (Saleebey, 1997).

3.3. Comparison of Different Theorists' Views on Spirituality

In comparing the different views of social scientists towards spirituality, it is notable that transpersonal theorists focus their studies on the whole person both inside and out including the body, mind, and spirit. Though the transpersonal theory is not easily tested, the application in counseling in clinical practice, especially in chronic illness and stress related issues, is increasing. To be named as the "fourth force" psychology by Maslow (1968), there is also increasing acceptance by other social scientists. However, many nontraditional approaches to growth and change including meditation, prayer, imagery, relaxation, and other mind-body or spiritual methods are still waiting for sufficient empirical support. In the psychoanalytic theory, the focus of study is on the unconsciousness, which is the inner world of a person. Since psychoanalysis is time consuming and psychoanalysts need longer time to develop one's expertise, there is not much clinical application. Though psychoanalytic theory is quite well accepted universally, its theory is difficult to be tested and there is a paucity of empirical study. Both Freud, the founder of the theory and Fromm, his follower, are negative towards spirituality. However, Jung, the Neo-Freudian, holds a different view from Freud and Fromm. In behavior approach, the focus of study is on observable behavior, which is mainly for the outer world. Since its theory is subject to rigorous testing, there are many empirical studies in this area. The clinical application and universal acceptance of the theory are strong. However, Skinner holds a very negative view towards spirituality that it is essentially subjective and difficult to be tested. Relating to the cognitive theories, the focus of the study is on the thinking process, which is the inner world of a person. Universal acceptance of the theory is strong with many clinical applications. Since this theory is also subject to tests, the number of empirical studies is also large. However, Ellis (1980) again holds a very negative view towards spirituality. For existential theory, the inner world is the focus for study. The logo-therapy developed by Frankl is quite well accepted by other social scientists with many clinical applications even though its theory is difficult to be tested with a paucity of empirical studies. Both Kierkegaard (1954) and Frankl (1963) are positive towards spirituality. Concerning the sociological theories, the functionalists such as Weber, Durkheim, and Parsons are positive towards spirituality/religion and recognize the important roles of religion in the society. On the other hand, Marx, adopting a conflict perspective of the society, is very resistive about religion. However, after the falling down of the Soviet Union, many communist countries are deserting Marxism and its universal acceptance is decreasing. A summary of the comparison of views on spirituality of different social scientists in terms of their basic dimensions is presented in Table 1.

Table 1. Comparison of views on spirituality of different social scientists in terms of their basic dimensions

Dimensions / Theories	Focus of study	Clinical application	Testability	Empirical studies	Universal acceptance	Views on spirituality
Transpersonal Maslow	Both inner and outer world	++	+	++	+	Positive
Psychoanalytic Freud Fromm Jung	Inner World	+	+	+	++	 Negative Negative Positive
Behavioral Skinner	Outer world	+++	+++	+++	+++	Negative
Cognitive Ellis	Inner world	+++	+++	+++	+++	Negative
Existential Kierkegarrd Frankl	Inner world	 + ++	 + +	 + +	 + ++	Positive
Functionalist Weber Durkheim Parsons	Outer world	++	+	+	++	Positive
Conflict Perspective Marx	Outer world	++	+	+	+	Negative
Strengths Perspective Saleebey	Both inner and outer world	++	+	+	+	Positive

Note: +++ strong; ++ medium; + weak

To summarize, there are negative and positive points of view towards spirituality and religion from different social scientists. Each has its argument that is worth paying attention to. However, no definite evidence has been found to support which side is much stronger than the other. This will be discussed in detail in the upcoming section. Therefore, an open mind should be maintained when investigating the spiritual dimension and this is also the approach adopted in this book.

Concerning the difference between spirituality/religion and social sciences, it has been suggested that as a science it has traditionally been regarded as a strictly objective, value-free description of behavior, so that subjective phenomena such as freedom of will, purpose, morality, and value, that are vital to religion are ultimately excluded from study (Marty, 1980). Under the dominance of positivism and the assumption that natural science methods of research are the only methods appropriate for a true science (Brennan, 1982; Cattell, 1947; Toulmin & Leary, 1985), religion is a topic that is most unlikely to be a candidate for scientific research. However, by the 1970s tension between the social sciences and religion had the chance to ease off, as a result of the erosion of the positivistic view of science. Kuhn (1970), the historian/philosopher of science, raised the importance of non-empirical considerations, such as the cultural and historical factors, values, worldviews, and language systems that shaped the scientific enterprise. Jones (1988) suggested, "...contemporary understandings of the nature of scientific knowledge and methods, by their explicit incorporation of non-empirical influences in their understanding of science, open the possibility that religious beliefs and commitments may have a valid role in the scientific process" (p. 142). The swing in behavioral science during the 1970s from the dominant, objective behaviorist doctrine to the subjective, cognitive and humanistic view was later called the cognitive, humanist or third revolution (Matson, 1971). It was a new perspective of understanding the world by taking the full range of people's inner experiences as legitimate for study. Such a paradigm shift, according to Sperry (1988), provides a holistic view to human science that has integrated the objective with the subjective data, the physical with the mental dimension, fact with value, and positivistic thought with phenomenology. Thus, with the acknowledgement of the importance of both the inner and outer world of the individual, it greatly enhances the possibility for integration between religion and social sciences.

Chapter 4

The Role of Spirituality in Nursing and Social Work Professionals

4.1. Definitions of Spirituality in Social Work

In social sciences literature, spirituality and religion have often been used interchangeably (Canda, 1988a, 1989) but also separately (Prest & Keller, 1993). However, as suggested by Canda (1997), the term "spirituality" was not used as commonly as the term "religion" during the early 1990s. The distinction between religion and spirituality is usually made with reference to religion as an association with an outward form of belief including rituals, dogmas, and denominational identity for religion; while spirituality refers to the inner feelings and experiences of the immediacy of a higher power (Bullis, 1996). They have in common the reference to a higher power, whether it is conceptualized within formal religious systems or not, or whether such a power is seen as God. Both, perhaps, express it as Lewis (1984) did in a central belief in an "invisible, personal, and living Spirit" (p. 451). Religious and spiritual experiences are manifested or mediated through rituals and other forms of communication-beliefs, such as myths, texts, emotions, and behaviors.

Spirituality is difficult to define since the concept is complex and different people might have different perceptions. The earliest attempt was made by Towle (1965) in "Common Human Needs," written primarily for social workers in public settings in the 1940s. She stated, "Spiritual needs of individual must be recognized, understood, and respected. Through the influence of religion the purpose of human life is better understood and sense of ethical values achieved" (pp. 6-11). However, the definition is not precise as there is no clear distinction between religion and spirituality. Later, formal attempts to develop a nonsectarian definition grew.

At present, the most commonly used definitions in current social work writing were established by Siporin (1985), Joseph (1987), and Canda (1988b). Siporin (1985) defined spiritual as, "a moral aspect of the person, called the soul, which is concerned about striving for transcendental values, a sense of meaning, knowledge of ultimate reality, and relatedness with other people and supernatural powers" (p. 199). He pointed out that spirituality might be expressed within or outside religious institutions. Joseph (1987), in discussing the religious and spiritual aspects of clinical practice in social work, defined religion as, "the external expression of one's faith, comprising beliefs, ethical codes, and worship which unite one to a moral community" (p. 14). Whereas faith he regarded as, "an internal system of beliefs and values which relates one to the transcendent or ultimate reality and orients one's life and behavior accordingly. For those with theistic beliefs, the ultimate reality is God" (p. 14). He further defined spirituality as "the underlying dimension of consciousness which strives for meaning, union with the universe, and with all things; it extends to the experience of the transcendent or a power beyond us. For believers, it includes one's relationship with and experience of God" (p. 14). Canda (1988b) sees spirituality as, "the human quest for personal meaning and mutually fulfilling relationships among people, the nonhuman environment, and, for some, God" (p. 243).

Despite attention for defining spirituality, there are still problems with the use of the concept in social work. One problem is the lack of consensus on precise meanings. However, two themes are reflected commonly in definitions given by practitioners in response to recent surveys (Derezotes & Evans, 1995; Sheridan & Bulis, 1991). First, spirituality is recognized as a natural part or capacity of all people involving a search for meaning. Second, spirituality as a basic aspect of human nature is distinguished from religion as an institution. Furthermore, O'Brien (1992) suggested that it is not necessary to have a consensus about a precise definition as long as a cluster of related themes are evoked by use of the concept. To name a few, some of his themes of spirituality included morality; the meaning and purpose of life; relation to ultimate reality; relations with nonphysical reality; the path to enlightenment or salvation, *etc*. For the working definition for this book, a broader sense of the definition from Joseph (1987) is adopted.

4.2. The Role of Spirituality in Nurses

Concerning the spiritual dimension of nursing, Bradshaw (1994) demonstrated that the roots of nursing were firmly fixed within a tradition of spiritual beliefs that were found, in her study, to be rooted within the Judeo-Christian tradition. Emerging nursing models developed by many nursing theorists addressed spirituality directly in terms of human needs (Newman, 1989; Rogers, 1970; Travelbee, 1971; Watson, 1985). Watson (1985) stated that nursing was emerging from a traditional practice of objective, rational detachment into something far greater. Part of that greatness included the renaissance of a holistic approach. As nursing redefines itself, it will reincorporate some of the forgotten aspects of the heritage - the role of the spirit. Watson (1988) further stated, "human caring theory allows the commitment and consciousness of the nurse to transcend (or at least attempt to transcend) the physical material surface and reach beyond to touch the human center of the person" (p. 176).

Meeting the spiritual needs of clients has become a recognized part of nursing in most of the western cultures. Nursing care is not only to make clients well or prevent illness, "but to help those in health or illness to use the power within themselves as they evolve toward higher levels of consciousness" (Rogers, 1970). One of the first empirical studies of nurses' spirituality conducted by Dennis (1991) suggested that spiritual care was not a separate part of nursing, but that it was integral to nursing, as evidenced by the range of comments supporting spirituality in practice.

In a qualitative study of the views of spiritual care by Conco (1995), findings revealed that spiritual care was given and received in a context in which the recipient was vulnerable and receptive to spiritual care. Three theme clusters included enabling transcendence of the present situation for higher meaning and purpose, enabling hope, and establishing connectedness. In the study by Coulon et al., (1996) on "the pursuit of excellence in nursing care", qualitative data showed that a holistic care approach to caring was one of the four major themes that emerged. In a pilot study to explore elderly patient perceptions of their spiritual needs and care by Ross (1997), the types of spiritual needs experienced were related to religion, meaning, love and belonging, morality, and death and dying. Ways in which they might be helped to meet their spiritual needs include enabling them to attend hospital services or providing a quiet room for prayer/reflection, as well as improving links with the chaplaincy service.

Spirituality is a complex concept. There are different definitions from different nursing authors. It has been described by Soeken and Carson (1987), as a belief that relates a person to the world, giving meaning to existence; a personal quest to find meaning and purpose in life (Burkhardt & Nagai-Jacobson, 1985); and a transcendental relationship or sense of connection with mystery, a higher being, God or Universe (Ellis, 1980; O'Brien, 1982). Spirituality within these definitions could refer to its narrow sense as a transcendental relationship to God and in its broad sense as a searching for meaning and purpose of life.

Carson (1989) suggested there was both a vertical and horizontal dimension to a person's spirituality. The vertical dimension deals with the person's transcendent (beyond and/or outside self) relationship with a higher being or God. The horizontal dimension reflects the supreme value of one's God through one's life. There is a continuous interrelationship between and among the inner being of the person, the person's vertical and horizontal dimensions with self, others, and the environment. The individual's relationships are based on expressions of love, forgiveness, and trust, and result in meaning and purpose in life.

The increasing interest of nursing in providing holistic care to clients has encouraged diverse approaches to the conceptualization and understanding of spirituality. Summarized by Carson (1989), three approaches have emerged in the interpretation of spirituality: spiritual distress (Carpenito, 1983), spiritual needs (Fish & Shelly, 1978; Highfield & Cason, 1983: stallwood & Stoll, 1975) and spiritual well-being (Cook, 1980; Ellison, 1983; Moberg, 1979; Paloutzian & Ellison, 1982). Each approach has its strengths and sheds light on a different facet of spirituality but they also complement one another in providing a more comprehensive picture.

Since Christianity is the national religion in most of the western countries, providing spiritual care is widely accepted. However, among the above approaches, spiritual distress as a "Nursing Diagnosis" is mostly used by nurses in U.S.A and Canada for providing nursing care. A nursing care plan is formulated after the "Nursing Diagnosis" is made. In Hong Kong, holistic care is one of the key elements when speaking of quality health care service and meeting a client's spiritual care is becoming a heated topic for discussion among all health care professionals. Position statements on holistic care have been published by the Nursing Section of the Hospital Authority in which the provision of spiritual care is much emphasized (Hospital Authority, 2001). In the statement, it is asserted that the needs of clients are beyond the physical aspect and the concept of holism is an important element for good quality of care. It further provides a framework including the environment, nursing system, client assessment, nursing competence, and caring process for the delivery of holistic care. It envisages that holistic care is crucial to quality nursing service and the outcomes will be positive from all parties concerned including clients, professionals, and the health care institutions. Finally, some guidelines in management, professional and personal development, clinical nursing practice, and research are recommended to practice holistic care for the benefits of both clients and staff. In the meantime, training to enhance meeting client's spiritual needs is conducted in some hospitals particularly those with a Christian background.

From nursing colleagues, some lessons could be learned in enlightening our practice of social work in Hong Kong. Firstly, the nursing professionals have the affirmation of the spiritual need of a whole person that gives the direction of providing nursing service in a holistic approach. Secondly, holistic nursing has been added into the curriculum of most of the nursing training, which enhances the understanding of the concept and the preparation of student nurses to put theory into practice when they finish their training. While in some hospitals, measures such as the design of the assessment form and nursing care plan have been taken in order to integrate the concept of spiritual care into practice complemented with in-service training on holistic care (e.g., Alice Ho Miu Ling Nethersole Hospital, 2002). Finally, research on spiritual care including the attitude of nursing staff, intervention, and outcomes are more encouraged. It is time for us, as social work professionals, to reflect our practice of holistic care in aspects of clinical practice, education, administration, and research using the nursing professionals as an example.

4.3. The Role of Spirituality in Social Work

Historical trends

Concerning the role of spirituality in social work, Canda (1997) outlined three historical phases in the United States. Phase 1 was the sectarian origins that began with the establishment of the American colonies through the first few decades of the 1900s. During that period, social work arose to a great extent out of sectarian institutions and ideologies pertaining to charity and community service. The most influential religious perspectives were Christian and Jewish. The second phase was from the professionalism and secularization of the 1920s through the 1970s. With the increasing pluralistic society, where religious composition changed dramatically, and the quest of scientific status that regarded religion as antithesis to science, religious based moralistic judgmentalism stimulating objection and avoidance of proselytizing, the profession tended to distance itself from its religion origins.In the late 1970s, the third phase, a resurgence of interest in spirituality began to emerge and had gained momentum rapidly since the 1980s. Beyond public interest concerning religious and spiritual issues, this phase was initiated with a few books about spiritual perspective on social work that went beyond the Judeo-Christian tradition, such as Brandon's Zen in the "Art of Helping" (1976) and Krill's "Existential Social Work" (1978). During the 1980s, many more publications called for attention to spirituality in an inclusive manner (Canda, 1988a, 1988b, 1989; Constable, 1983; Joseph, 1987, 1988; Marty, 1980; Meystedt, 1984; Siporin, 1982, 1985). During the 1990s, research on spirituality and social work continued to grow, focusing more on specific practice and education issues (Boyd, 1998; Canda & Phaobtong, 1992; Carroll, 1997; Cowley, 1993; Cowley & Derezotes, 1994; Saleebey, 1997; Sermabeikian, 1994; Sheridan et al., 1992; Sheridan, Wilmer & Atcheson, 1994; Tan, 1996). The first social work practice textbook focusing on spirituality from a nonsectarian perspective was published in 1996 (Bullis, 1996). Bullis reported empirical data on the use of spiritual and religious practices by clinical social workers. Using clear, cogent, and specific examples of interventions, the book also considered advocacy and public policy issues. Accompanying increasing numbers of publication, there were growing numbers of presentations on spirituality and religious diversity at national conferences and professional networking through the National Association of Social Workers (NASW), Council of Social Work Education (CSWE), and other organizations from the mid-1980s onwards. The 1995 version of the CSWE's Handbook of Accreditation Standards and Procedures provided a clear indicator of this professional shift. Important areas of curriculum content such as belief systems, religion, and spirituality were mentioned with special attention to the diversity among clients (Russel, 1998). In NASW's 2001 Standard for Culture Competence in Social Work Practice, it strongly advised practitioners to meet their clients' spiritual needs and the 2008 Code of Ethics of the NASW also stipulated addressing their clients' religion as a standard of practice (Hodge & Horvath, 2011).

The relevance of spirituality/religion in social work

For the past few decades, studies of the relevance of spirituality/religion in social work have been increasing. Using the terms "spirituality" and "religion" to search the number of publications in Social Work Abstracts, there were 210 and 381 numbers of records, during the years 1977 to 2003, respectively. Some representative articles in chronological order were illustrated for discussion. In the 1980s, studies such as Constable (1983) demonstrating the religious roots of the social work practice, Cox (1983) examining the role of religion in the delivery of welfare services to immigrants, Meystedt (1984) finding a prominent role religion played in rural life, and Siporin (1986) discussing the contribution of religious values to social work, all showed the significant influence of spirituality/religion in social work.

In the 1990s, more empirical studies had been conducted on spirituality and religion. Suggestions had been made by social work educators to include the religious/spiritual dimension into social work education, and social workers were urged to integrate spirituality and religion into their clinical practice. Canda (1991) argued that there was an inadequacy of the western developmental theories in addressing the spiritual dimensions of human behavior and asserted that transpersonal theory could provide a more holistic perspective in working with Asians and non-Asians alike. A study by Sheridan et al., (1992) of 328 randomly selected clinicians including social workers, psychologists, and counselors found that a majority of them used religious or spiritual interventions in working with their clients. The authors concluded as a whole, respondents were found to value the religious or spiritual dimension in their own lives and to some extent to address them in their practice. However, 79% of them reported that religious and spiritual issues were not addressed during their training and education. A survey by Sheridan, Wilmer, and Atcheson (1994) showed that the majority (82.5%) of the full time social work educators supported the inclusion of the topic of religion and spirituality in the social work curriculum, though primarily as an elective.

Bergin (1991) suggested three major contributions to therapy arising from a spiritual perspective.

Conception of human nature

A spiritual reality and the spiritual experiences can make a difference in a person's behavior, thus influencing one's identity, agency, and life-style.

Studies show that there are relations between spiritual experiences and observable behaviors that reflect mental status and life-styles (Bergin, Masters & Richards, 1987; Bergin et al., 1988); and spiritual conviction and physical health (Antonovsky, 1979; Martin & Carlson, 1988; McIntosh & Spilka, 1990). Hence, the spiritual experiences facilitate the study of significant psychological phenomena.

Moral frame of reference

A spiritual perspective could provide a moral frame of reference and emphasize that therapy is not value free because it views the world in value-laden terms. It also helps therapists feel more confident about value choices that can be used as cognitive guides to their clients' life-styles.

Techniques

A spiritual perspective provides a set of techniques (e.g., Collins, 1980) ranging from intra-psychic methods to family and social system methods: the use of prayer, scripture study, and rituals such as worship and communal spiritual experience. Another technique, which has been shown to be successful is the transitional figure method described in detail by Bergin et al., (1988). Studies also show that religious rituals are therapeutic. For example, Griffith & Young (1988) found that the Christian religious ritual in black churches could offer participants security, support, and identity.

Canda and Phaobtong (1992) noted that the social structures of Buddhist temples were resources for Southeast Asian refugees. Social workers were advised to use them as reference points to provide culturally sensitive services for this population. Abramovitz (1993) reported that daily ritual prayer among frail Jewish elderly provided a positive orientation for day program attendees, which was ultimately therapeutic. Sermabeikian (1994), using Jung's analytic psychology as a theoretical framework for understanding spirituality within the individual, proposed that the acknowledgment of their clients' spiritual beliefs and values would contribute to the therapeutic benefits of intervention. Taggart (1994), a clinical social worker with theological background, strongly advocated the relevance of spirituality in clinical practice. She argued that it was imperative to explore one's belief system that affected one's thinking, feeling, and action. Religious belief that defines a universal meaning to human life and usually implies some sort of deity is one of the belief systems for some people. Therefore, we have to explore the client's religious beliefs, as well as any other beliefs. She further suggested that a religious belief system defined what was real and good, which provided one with direction and purpose of life. She also recommended the use of a journal, meditation, and religious support groups in one's clinical practice. Natural Support Systems represent an important community resource for meeting Puerto Rican elder's social service needs. In a study of 558 Puerto Rican elders, 214 of which indicated having a functional disability, Delgado (1996) found that religion was widely considered the second most important support beyond that of the family.

Towards the 21st century, for many clients, there is a growing realization that spirituality is a personal strength that can be operationalized in clinical settings to lessen problems (Ai, 2000; Carroll, 1997; Pargament, 1997; Richards & Bergin, 1997). The diversity of the beneficial relationships spirituality engenders is also extensive. The positive effects could be found in different stages of a personal life span. Especially, during the late life when people tends to face more negative life events in coping with the reality of chronic conditions, disabilities, losses, and death. Various measures of spirituality are positively associated with: interpersonal friendliness (Ellison, 1992), satisfying marriages (Kaslow & Robison, 1996), resiliency (Haight, 1998), coping (Pargament, 1997), and successful aging (Kimble et al., 1995). It has also been associated with decreased rates of substance abuse (Benson, 1992), recovery from divorce (Nathanson, 1995), and sexual assault (Kennedy, Davis, & Talyor, 1998).

Building upon existing theory and research, Hodge (2000a) developed a theoretical framework of spirituality. The framework delineates seven pathways through which spirituality fosters individual change in five salutary outcomes. The seven pathways are: health promotive behaviors and lifestyles, social support, psychodynamics of ritual, psychodynamics of cognitive schemata, ego challenge, quantum effects, and supernatural effects. The five salutary outcomes are: decreased alcohol, tobacco and other drug usage, decreased morbidity and mortality, increased resiliency and coping, increased pro-social attitudes and behaviors, and increased mental health. The author suggested the framework could provide a theoretical road map for workers to understand, and utilize consumers' spiritual resources.

Though many studies show the positive effects of religion and spirituality to both individual and collective behaviors, other studies indicate some negative influences of religion on behavior. Wikler (1986) found that some orthodox Jews might attach a sense of stigma and community sanction, such as damage to family reputation or reduced marriage prospects to people with mental illness. They tended to refrain from utilizing mental health services. Furthermore, many orthodox rabbis might not refer people who could benefit from mental health services to mental institutions. In studying families with critically ill infants in the neonatal intensive care unit, York (1987) found some families using a harmful form of religious denial to deal with treatment decisions – a belief in miracles that their infants might not need treatment in their recovery by withholding treatment.

There has been concern about the professional intervention on client's values especially on religious issues. Meadow (1986) expressed the worry of including religion in therapy by those therapists with limited knowledge of religion. However, Meadow's concern is perhaps not substantiated as it has been demonstrated that values are constantly at play in therapy, and that clinicians would apply his/her certain values during therapy and try to develop them in their clients (Bergin, 1980; Bergin, 1985; London, 1986; Strupp, Hadley, & Gomes-Schwartz, 1977). As commented by Bergin (1991), when making important decisions about how to enhance clients' function, therapists have to base the treatment on their professional values, which are frequently implicit. It is suggested the more explicit this valuational process, the more likely the client could make his/her individual value choices, which leads to more collaboration between therapist and client with agreed upon goals for change. Prest and Keller (1993) noted that during psychotherapy, on some level the metaphysical beliefs of the practitioner were always being shared. Hodge (1998) argued that the question was no longer whether values would be communicated in therapeutic settings, but what type of framework would be conveyed. The issue was what Thompson (1990) argued, how to use values to a therapeutic advantage without violating the client's self-determination. A study by Hodge (2000b) showed that client's self-determination was valued both in faith-based and secular residential treatment programs.

Based upon a post-modern perspective that all organizations conveyed a particular set of values, and clients would tend to select programs congruent with their pre-existing metaphysical values, Hodge (2000b) explored the relationship between faith-based providers and autonomy by comparing perceptions of autonomy at two privately funded, faith-based residential programs with those of two comparable, government-funded, secular programs. The two faith-based residential programs for substance abuse treatment, with integration of their specific convictions into every aspect of the program through regularly scheduled scripture study, praise times, etc. were selected because all staff were Christian; Christian spirituality was the primary therapeutic intervention. The other two programs were generally secular in orientation, adhering to no specific metaphysical framework. The survey instrument consisted of 56 questions measuring perceptions of self-determination within a program, the degree of congruency between consumers' metaphysical beliefs prior to program selection, and their chosen programs, spiritual values and practices, and religious beliefs. A response rate was 58% with 116 questionnaires returned (n=68 clients, n=48 staff). The study suggested that faith-based providers might have the same degree of respect for client autonomy as equivalent secular service providers. Thus, it implied that clients found their right to self-determination to be equally valued in faith-based and secular programs.

Recently, the strengths perspective with the integration of the spiritual dimension is becoming popular in social work practice. A framework of strengths perspective with the application of five themes from the Chinese philosophical tradition of Taoism, which integrates the spiritual dimension, was proposed by Koneig and Spano (1998) as a guide for social work practice. A qualitative study conducted by Canda (2002) on the significance of spirituality for resilient response to chronic illness (n=16), showed that spirituality was a source of strength supporting health and well-being. The study also highlighted the need of social workers to address spirituality as strength in adversity, such as facing chronic illness and disability. However, a review of the empirical studies by Staudt, Howard, and Drake (2001) showed that few evaluations of strength-based treatment have been published and there is still not enough support for the strengths perspective as a distinct and uniquely effective practice model.

To sum up, there are increasing evidences to support the relevance of spirituality/religion in social work. Furthermore, there is a close relationship of religion with social work; we could see that religion has shared the same concern of social work for alleviating human suffering. A religious and spiritual perspective to social work offers additional therapeutic techniques such as prayer, rituals, and supporting groups to those clients who do not have religious beliefs. It would be more effective to those clients with religious background, since they are familiar with the additional therapeutic techniques arising out of their religious practices.

Chapter 5

EMPIRICAL STUDIES INVESTIGATING THE ROLE OF SPIRITUALITY IN TREATMENT

Though, the rise of the holistic healing movement in the west started only during the end of the last century, academics and healthcare professionals had carried out a number of empirical studies investigating the role of spirituality. Some studies by healthcare professionals were summarized in chronological order and presented as follows.

5.1. RESEARCH BY MEDICAL PROFESSIONALS

Series of cases have suggested acupuncture, the approach of one tradition, Chinese medicine, may be effective as either a primary or adjunctive treatment in a variety of psychiatric, as well as psycho-physiologic disorders (Chen, 1979; Shanghai College of Traditional Medicine, 1981). The capacity of acupuncture to alter central nervous system physiology and biochemistry, including most particularly the release of a variety of neurotransmitters, endorphins, and encephalin, has been repeatedly demonstrated (Stux & Pomeranz, 1987).

A study by Shapiro (1982) showed that meditative techniques of the various spiritual traditions could bring about a generalized reduction in many physiological systems, thereby creating a state of relaxation. He further noted that "this state" could not be "differentiated from the effects of other relaxation techniques whether they be hypnosis or deep muscle relaxation" (p. 269).

In a study of prayer as a kind of spiritual intervention, Byrd (1988) used a double-blind, 2 parallel groups design for 393 coronary care patients. Prayer, in Christian tradition, was used as an experimental intervention. 3 to 7 intercessors were assigned per patient until the patient was released from the hospital. The intercessors were required to have an active Christian life with daily devotional prayer and active participation in a local church. On the other hand, usual care was performed in the control group. It was found that the group receiving intercessory prayer had an overall better outcome, requiring less antibiotics, diuretics, and intubations /ventilation than the control group.

In everyday practice, some general practitioners accept the idea of spiritual healing as a positive source of patient well-being and incorporate spiritual healing into their practice (by laying on of hands, or praying with patients), or include spiritual healers as part of their referral network (Cohen, 1989; Pietroni, 1986).

Koenig et al.,(1992) studied 850 elderly hospitalized men and found those religious behaviors such as prayer, the reading of scriptures, or having a strong faith in God protected older medically-ill patients against the emotional stresses of hospitalization, as well as acute illnesses. Koenig and Weaver (1997) had shown an important relationship between religious commitment and positive mental health status among the elderly. Koenig (1997) found that many seniors who practiced their faith had lower levels of depression, anxiety, and alcoholism; higher life satisfaction and greater well-being; and adapted better to the rigors of personal loss, physical illness, and disability.

Sicher et al.,(1998) conducted a double blind, 2 parallel groups of different distant healing methods for 40 patients with AIDS. In the experimental group, distant healing was used as intervention. 40 healers from different spiritual traditions were recruited. Each patient was treated by 10 healers. The control group was treated with the usual care. Results showed that the experimental group had fewer new AIDS-defining illnesses, less illness severity, fewer physician visits and hospitalizations, and improved mood.

With a double blind, 2 parallel groups design, Harris et al.,(1999) studied 990 coronary care patients. Remote intercessory prayer in Christian tradition was used for experimental intervention for 28 days per patient. However, qualifications for being an intercessor were different from Byrd's in that they were not required to have any particular denominational affiliation. Furthermore, they needed to agree with the beliefs that God is concerned with individual lives and is responsive to prayers for healing made on behalf of the sick. Usual care was performed in the control group. Results showed that there were significant effects for summed and weighted coronary care unit score but no differences in length of hospital stay.

In a meta-analysis of randomized controlled trials on the clinical effect of Qigong practice on essential hypertension, Guo et al.,(2008) found that self-practiced qigong for less than 1 year is better in decreasing blood pressure in patients with essential hypertension than in no-treatment controls, but is not superior to active controls in which qigong is combined with drug treatments.

Not all studies on holistic care have positive results. Some studies on the treatment modalities in holistic medicine have been found with no effect. However, adverse effects in holistic care are rarely found. Astin et al.,(2000) conducted a systematic review of the available data on the efficacy of any form of "distant healing" including prayer, mental healing, Therapeutic Touch or spiritual healing as treatment for any medical condition. A total of 23 trials involving 2,774 patients met the inclusion criteria and were analyzed. Of the trials, five examined prayer as the distant healing intervention, eleven assessed noncontact Therapeutic Touch, and seven examined other forms of distant healing. Among the 23 studies, 13(57%) yielded statistically significant treatment effects, 9 showed no effect over control interventions, and 1 showed a negative effect. Though there were methodological limitations in several studies, which made it difficult to draw definitive conclusions, the findings indicated that approximately 57% of trials showed a positive treatment effect and the evidence supported further study.

Abbot et al.,(2001) conducted a randomized clinical trial to study the efficacy of healing in the treatment of chronic pain. One hundred and twenty patients suffering from chronic pain that were resistant to conventional treatments were recruited from a Pain Management Clinic. The trial had two parts: face-to-face healing or simulated face-to-face healing for 30 minutes per week for 8 weeks (part I); and distant healing or no healing for 30 minutes per week for 8 weeks (part II). The McGill Pain Questionnaire, VAS for pain, SF36, Hospital Anxiety and Depression scale, and a patient profile were used for outcome measures. Outcome measures were obtained before, then after 3 and 8 weeks of the trial. The findings showed that subjects in healing groups, in both parts I and II, reported significantly more 'unusual experiences' during the sessions, but the clinical relevance of that was unclear. The study concluded that a specific effect of face-to-face or distant healing on chronic pain could not be demonstrated over eight treatment sessions in these patients.

Benson et al.,(2006) conducted a randomized clinical trial on the effects of intercessory prayer on 1,802 cardiac patients undergoing surgery in 6 hospitals, whom were randomly assigned to 3 different groups. Results showed that no differences between the outcomes of subjects who received prayer and subjects who did not receive prayer. Furthermore, it was found that patients who were told to receive prayer did worse than others, though the statistically significant difference was small.

With the increasing evidence in the medical literature that suggests a strong relationship between spirituality and medicine, more attention is paid on the assessment of the spiritual needs of patients. Knowing that 40% of patients expected physicians should discuss pertinent religious issues but only 11% of physician always did, Anadarajah and Hight (2001) developed a teaching tool "HOPE", which are questions to help medical students, residents, and practicing physicians incorporate spiritual assessment into the medical interview. The HOPE questions cover four basic areas of inquiry for physicians in formal spiritual assessments. They are as follows: H-sources of hope, strength, comfort, meaning, peace, love and connection; O-the role of organized religion for the patient; P-personal spirituality and practices; E-effects on medical care and end-of-life decisions. Though the tool has not been validated by research, it provides a comprehensive guide to explore an individual's general spiritual resources and needs.

A surgeon usually emphasizes on the physical need of a patient and justifies his or her position by accurate diagnosis and surgical operation skill. Hinshaw (2002) advocated that surgeons should include more than addressing the patient's physical ill. He used two case examples to demonstrate the importance of spiritual needs of a dying patient and recommended two tools, "a spiritual history" and "a patient's biography" for spiritual assessment. Skills for spiritual intervention were also discussed.

In the early twentieth century, not much was taught about spirituality or religion in the medical schools in the United States. According to the American Medical Association, the number of medical schools offering courses on religion and spiritual issues has been increasing. It is estimated approximately 70% of all medical schools have courses on spirituality or religion and medicine at present (Puchalski, 2006).

5.2. Research by Nursing Professionals

A best known clinical study by Krieger (1975) demonstrated significant increases in the hemoglobin values of a group of patients who had been touched by nurses trained to enter a meditative state and experience their "healing intention" toward their patients. Wirth et al.,(1993) used a double blind randomized, placebo-controlled trial of Therapeutic Touch for 24 participants with experimentally induced puncture wounds. In the experimental group, non-contact Therapeutic Touch was performed by a healer behind a one-way mirror 5 minutes per day for 10 days. In the control group, no treatment was done. It was found that there was more rapid healing in the treatment group. Gordon et al.,(1998) used a single blind randomized, controlled trial of Therapeutic Touch for 31 patients with osteoarthritis of the knee. In the experimental group, non-contact Therapeutic Touch was performed 1 session per week for 6 weeks. In the control group, mock therapeutic touch and usual care were performed. It was found that the treatment group showed improvements in pain, health status, and function. Turner et al.,(1998) conducted a single blind, 2 parallel groups for 99 burn patients. In the experimental group, non-contact Therapeutic Touch was performed for 5 days with time varied from 5 to 20 minutes. In the control group, mock Therapeutic Touch was done instead. A positive effect was found in the experimental group with reductions in pain and anxiety.

Reed (1987), in a study of spirituality and well-being in terminally ill hospitalized patients, found that for the terminally ill patients, there was indeed a shift toward greater spirituality as indicated by a stronger faith and increased prayer. Adults who become increasingly aware of their own mortality appear to develop a greater need for the spiritual dimension of life.

In a study by Sutton and Murphy (1989), 40 patients with less than 4 years after a kidney transplant rated the extent to which they used each of the 40 coping strategies to deal with stress. It was found that prayer and looking at the problem objectively were used most often in coping with stress. Saudia et al.,(1991) examined the relationship between a sense of control over one's own health and the helpfulness of prayer as a direct-action coping mechanism in patients about to have cardiac surgery. The result showed that prayer was perceived as a helpful, direction-action coping mechanism.

In a qualitative study conducted by Sullivan (1993), 40 respondents with chronic and severe psychiatric disabilities were interviewed. 48% of them reported that spiritual beliefs and practices were essential to their success in coping and recovery. In a study by Lindgren and Coursey (1995), it was found that 83% of their sample of individuals who regularly attended a psychosocial rehabilitation center felt that their spiritual beliefs had a positive impact on the disability. In a related study, Kinsella, Anderson and Anderson (1996) found that 5 out of 20 adult offspring and siblings of individuals with a psychiatric disability specifically reported that a religious or spiritual faith was an important means of coping during their most difficult times.

In studying the spiritual dimension in patient care, Hawley and Irurita (1998) found that all praying gave participants comfort. The participants believed that God listened to their prayers and answered them when they were seeking comfort. It was this reassurance that gave them the strength to face uncertainty and possible death, and also gave them comfort in their psycho-physiological condition at the time. Besides, some studies also support that the caring of the spiritual dimension of the patient may have a better effect to the patient's outcome.

Pullen et al.,(1999) investigated relationships between alcohol and drug abuse by adolescents and frequency of religious service attendance in the southeast United States. Data collected from surveys of 217 adolescents, age 12-19 years, was analyzed. The adolescents included participants from both clinical and non-clinical settings. Results from both groups showed that, as attendance at religious services increased, alcohol and drug abuse decreased. They suggest spirituality is a concept that warrants further study to determine if its inclusion in treatment programs could enhance recovery or drastically reduce recidivism.

Chiu (2000) investigated the experience of spirituality in Taiwanese women with breast cancer through in-depth interviews with 15 women. Four main categories were developed based on a review of the interview transcripts. They were: living reality; creating meaning; connectedness; and transcendence. These not only helped understand the client's subjective experience about spirituality as a cancer patient but also enrich our understanding of the meaning of spirituality.

Pierce (2001) conducted an ethnographic study of caring and expressions of spirituality by urban caregivers of people with stroke in African-American families. Eight key informants (primary caregivers) and 16 general informants (secondary caregivers) were recruited in the study. After analysis of the data obtained from interviews, eight themes concerning spirituality for all caregivers were discovered: caring was viewed as a filial ethereal value, self-contemplation, motivation for philosophical introspection, filial piety, living in the moment and hope for the future, purpose, motivated by approval from care recipients, and Christian piety.

Shih et al.,(2001) presented the content outline of the first spiritual care program in a nursing degree for Master of Science students (N=22) in Taiwan, and also evaluated its usefulness in helping students provide spiritual care in various clinical settings. Results showed that all participants considered the spiritual care course to be helpful in assisting them to provide spiritual care for their clients in various clinical settings.

Cox (2003) used two case studies to illustrate how nurses could perform non-denominational spiritual interventions without compromising the belief systems of the client or nurse and without a great deal of material resources or time. This study suggests spiritual intervention may reduce clients' anxieties, leading to reduced dissatisfactions with care and facilitating client recovery and rehabilitation.

Koslander and Arridsson (2006) conducted a qualitative study by interviewing 12 psychiatric patients on their conceptions of how the spiritual dimension is addressed in mental health care. The findings revealed that patients wished to have their spiritual needs addressed. However, they lacked confidence in the nurses with regard to discussing spirituality and perceived that the nurses lacked knowledge about the spiritual dimension and avoided addressing their spiritual needs. In order to address their own spiritual needs, they turned to themselves and other patients for help.

An overview of the research done by the nursing profession on spiritual care in nursing between 1983 and 2005 was conducted by Ross (2006). Some essential components of spiritual care and related factors were identified. Results also showed that nurses received little education on the spiritual dimension of care and the need for further nursing education in spiritual care is highlighted.

A critical review on private prayer as a suitable intervention for hospitalized patients from totaling 26 qualitative and correlational studies was conducted by Hollywell and Walker, (2006). Results indicated that private prayer, when measured by frequency, is usually associated with lower levels of depression and anxiety. Samples with strong Christian traditions and a relatively high level of religiosity, church attendance, and use of prayer show positive associations between prayer and wellbeing.

5.3. Research by Social Work and Allied Health Professionals

Allied health professionals are those professional staff members beyond doctors and nurses in the healthcare team including mostly medical social workers, psychologists, occupational therapists, physiotherapists, and chaplains. In working with the elderly, Koenig, George, and Siegler (1988) discovered that in a sample of 100 elderly, aged 55 to 80, in responding to stressful life changes, 45% of them used religious coping behavior. Wilson

(1992), when working with rural black elderly women in North Carolina, found that to devise an effective health care program for the elderly, the program had to be embedded in the black church. Abramowitz (1993) found that there was a therapeutic value in prayer when it was included in a daily program for the mentally impaired Jewish elderly clients in Israel. In facing the death of an elderly parent, Scharlach and Fuller (1994) found that religion was one of the helpful coping resources for a group of adults, especially for the daughters. A literature review by Donahue and Benson (1995) indicated that adolescent religious involvement was positively associated with pro-social values, and negatively related to at risk behaviors including suicide, substance abuse, delinquency, premature sexual activity, and adolescent pregnancy.

In the area of social work intervention, Breton (1989) found that for engaging the poor and the oppressed, liberation theology in Latin America could provide ideas for social group workers. Whereas, in family therapy, Prest and Keller (1993) suggested to integrate spirituality into family therapy by increasing openness to address relevant spiritual beliefs, and metaphors in therapy, which could often provide the therapist with a more effective intervention. Nakhaima (1994) found that a family's church or religious community was a valuable resource in marital and family counseling but it had too often been overlooked. He further suggested a new model in family counseling that incorporated both religion and the natural family system in the counseling effort.

Klass's (1992) study showed the experiential and social dimensions of religion, particularly in the area of generating solace in bereaved parents, in a ten-year ethnographic study of a religious self-help group for parents who had lost a child. One of the means for relieving parental grief was by ritualizing the memory of the lost child yearly in a holiday candlelight memorial service. In conclusion, Klass urged the clergy to develop solace-supporting liturgies and suggested mental health professionals to re-examine their models of grief by taking notice of the healing potential of people's religious faith.

In working with religious clients, Propst (1980) reported more effectiveness of religious over non-religious imagery in treating mildly depressed cases. Lewis and Lewis (1985) found that religious clients were rated by therapists as requiring significantly fewer therapy sessions than their non-religious clients, independent of whether the therapists had a religious background or not. Gartner, Larson, and Allen's (1991) study on religion and mental health, also showed that clients who participated in religious activities and religiously-based psychotherapeutic interventions, tended to have better improvement in psychological functioning.

In the study by Maton (1989), it is believed that spiritual support, like social support, can have beneficial stress-reducing effects. Maton suggests that spiritual support operates through two pathways: cognitive mediation and emotional support. Cognitive mediation refers to the positive interpretation and "appraisal of the meaning and implications of negative life events" (p. 311). The emotional support pathway includes the "perception of being valued, loved, and cared for by God" (p. 311). Pargament (1997) suggests that religion, as a coping mechanism serves five essential purposes. Firstly, spiritually it provides a sense of personal closeness with God, as well as meaning, purpose, and hope. Secondly, for self-development, it helps in feeling good about one's self and being more in control. Thirdly, it resolves self-efficacy and produces a sense of peace and comfort. Fourthly, it offers closeness, connectedness to a community, and meets intimacy needs. Finally, it helps in keeping emotions and behavior under control. Based on extensive empirical data, he concluded that religion appeared to be more helpful to some disadvantaged groups, such as the elderly, poor, less educated, blacks, widowed, and women. One of the reasons was because secular resources were less tangible to them while religion had become a viable alternative.

In a recent study, Ng and Shek (2001) examined the role of religion in therapy by investigating changes of 86 Chinese heroin-addicted men from different stages of a gospel drug rehabilitation program. It was found that there were positive changes in terms of less depressive and hopelessness symptoms, and a greater sense of purpose in life.

Hodge (2001) introduced a new qualitative spiritual-assessment instrument for social work practitioners after reviewing the existing qualitative assessment tools. The instrument consists of two components. The first part is an initial narrative framework to elicit a client's spiritual history. The second part is an interpretive framework to elicit a client's spiritual strength. The instrument would help social work practitioners assess their client's spirituality and elicit untapped strength.

Jorm et al., (2002) conducted a systematic review on the effectiveness of complementary and self-help treatments for depression. Data sources were from a systematic literature search using PubMed, PsycLit, the Cochrane Library, and previous review papers. Results showed that there was some limited evidence to support the effectiveness of Complementary medicine such as acupuncture, massage therapy, yoga breathing exercises, etc. They concluded that although none of the treatments reviewed were not as well supported by evidence as standard treatments, such as antidepressants and cognitive behavior therapy, many warranted further research.

Chamiec-Case (2009) using focus groups, individual interviews, and expert judges, developed an instrument to measure the extent to which social workers perceive that they integrate spirituality in the workplace. The field test survey of 745 respondents of a 21-item, 3 subscales version of the "Integration of Spirituality in the Workplace", showed good reliability and validity. This study also provides solid evidence that many social workers do in fact perceive that they integrate their spirituality in their work.

Hodge and Horvath (2011) used a qualitative meta-synthesis (N=11 studies) to identify and describe clients' perceptions of their spiritual needs in health care settings. The study showed 6 interrelated themes including meaning, purpose and hope; relationship with God; spiritual practices; religious obligations; inter-personal connection; and professional staff interaction. The results helped equip practitioners with a better spiritual knowledge to meet their clients' needs.

The above studies showed some positive evidence of the therapeutic values of the spiritual or religious dimension in helping people. Rare negative evidence was found so far. One possible reason is that most of the alternative treatments are physically harmless (Fergusson, 1995). Furthermore, research with negative results might not be submitted for publication. Nevertheless, from the accumulation of the increasing positive evidence at present, it warrants our attention to seriously consider having religious input in social work intervention. But, there are not many studies in this area of social work, particularly in psychiatric rehabilitation.

Chapter 6

The Importance of Spiritual Dimension in Psychiatric Rehabilitation

6.1. Spirituality/Religion and Mental Health

Some previous surveys demonstrated that religious and spiritual issues were often addressed in psychotherapy. In a survey of member psychologists of the American Psychiatric Association by Shafranske and Maloney (1990), 60% reported that clients often expressed their personal experiences in religious language and that at least one in six of their patients presented issues that directly involved religion or spirituality. Another study of psychologists by Lannert (1991) showed that 72% had at some time addressed religious or spiritual issues in treatment. In a survey by Bergin and Jensen (1990) with samples including psychologists, psychiatrists, social workers, and marriage and family therapists, 29% agreed that religious issues were important in the treatment of all or many of their clients. With the similarity of religious issues in those who sought help from mental health professionals, questions had been raised about the effect of religion on one's mental health.

Empirical research showed contradictory findings about the relationship between religion and mental health. On the one hand, evidence showed that some forms of religion were linked with emotionally and mentally unhealthy characteristics and behaviors. On the other hand, substantial evidence also showed that there was no necessary connection between religion and emotional disturbance. That in fact, many highly religious people were mentally healthy individuals. In a number of empirical studies, religious and non-religious individuals were found to have similar normal psychological and developmental characteristics. A comprehensive paper of previous reviews (1958-1991) of the relationship between religion/spirituality and mental health by Schumaker (1992) demonstrated this controversial picture. Some previous representative reviews on the positive side are discussed.

Argyle and Beit-Hallahmi (1975/1958) reviewed the studies on religion and personal adjustment, and concluded that religion was positively associated with measures of personal adjustment. The reasons might be religious participation could offer support, companionship, and a sense of identity and belonging to the participants. When studying whether religion could function as an effective coping mechanism during crisis, it appeared overall to be marginally helpful, since not many people turn to the church for help when in time of crisis, though they might resort to prayer. Some evidence showed that religious involvement was associated with lower rates of suicide and also played a role in the control of impulsive behavior, including alcohol consumption.

Lea's review (1982) summarized the previous two decades of research with mostly the correlational nature of studies mainly on student groups or religious groups as samples. The conclusions were drawn as follows: 1) for students, religiosity was related to personal inadequacy, but for adults, especially the elderly, it was associated positively to adjustment; 2) religiosity was not related to either social deviancy or moral behavior; 3) "healthy" religion was marked by "social responsibility, and relatedness to other parts of life and to a being greater than oneself, however defined" (p. 347); and 4) "unhealthy" religion involved a pre-occupation with guilt-generating concerns (e.g., sin, evil), and "rigidity with respect to healthy sexual and emotional functioning, and idiosyncratic and literal interpretation of religious symbolism" (p. 347).

Batson and Ventis' (1982) review found that the relationship between religion and mental health changes according to one's definition of mental health. Religion tended to have a positive effect on mental health when defined as the absence of psychological symptoms. But was more likely associated with impaired psychological functioning when defined with reference to personal competence, self-actualization, and flexibility, which highlighted the multi-dimensional nature of the concept of religion. This review also explored religion in terms of intrinsic, extrinsic, and quest orientation. The extrinsic orientation, roughly equivalent to immature religion, consists of using religion to gain some end, such as emotional or social support or social status. Intrinsic orientation (mature religion) consists of experiencing religion as a master motive in one's life that is internalized and fully lived (Allport & Ross, 1967). Intrinsic religiousness is positively correlated with the seven mental health criteria: absence of mental illness symptoms, appropriate social behavior, freedom from worry and guilt, personal competence and control, self-acceptance and self-actualization, unification and organization, and open-mindedness and flexibility. Besides, it is a generally positive force in the three broad areas of psychological adjustment, social conduct, and mental health (Payne et al., 1991). Whereas, extrinsic religiousness, is negatively associated with the seven mental health criteria and acts as an impediment in the three general areas.

The systematic review by Gartner et al.,(1991), consisting of over 200 studies, found that about half of which indicated a positive association and less than a quarter of which pointed to negative effects of religion. They also concluded that religiousness has a beneficial association with suicide risk, drug use, alcohol abuse, delinquent behavior, divorce and marital satisfaction, psychological well-being, depression, and physical health and longevity.

Some previous representative reviews of possible negative relationships between religion and mental health are also discussed as follows:

Dittes (1969) associated religion with personal inadequacy, intellectual inadequacy, hyper-suggestibility, and "desperate and generally unadaptive defensive maneuvers" (p. 636). By analyzing several studies dealing with religion and self-esteem, he argued that religion was "correlated with indices of pathology and deficiency" (p. 637). Suggestibility was seen by Dittes to mean a general personal weakness, an inhibition of personal initiative, submissiveness to authority, and a stagnant to an institutional religion.

Sanua's research review showed that there was no convincing evidence to support correlation between religiousness and mental health. On the subject of religion and psychological adjustment, Sanua (1969) concluded, "Most studies show no relationship between religiousness and mental health, while others point out that the religious person may at times show greater anxiety and at times less anxiety" (p. 1206). With regard to deviancy and social pathology, he summarized his view as follows, "The evidence regarding the relationship between social pathology and religion points out that the latter may not necessarily fulfill the function ascribed to it – namely, that of an integrating force in society and a contributor to the mental health of the members of that society" (p. 1207).

The review by Gartner et al.,(1991) also concluded that religion was related negatively to authoritarianism, self-actualization, suggestibility/

dependency, temporal lobe epilepsy, and dogmatism/tolerance of ambiguity/rigidity.

Concerning these contradictory findings, some researchers suggested it reflects the variety of ways of defining and measuring religion and mental health. A pattern noted is that negative relationships between religion and mental health tend to occur when "soft" or intra-psychic measures of mental health (e.g., paper-and-pencil instruments with authoritarianism) are used, whereas positive relationships tend to occur when "hard" or behavioral variables are used (e.g., measures of drug use, rates of delinquency) (Bergin, 1983; Donahue, 1985; Gartner et al., 1991; Schumaker, 1992).

Bergin (1983) provided a meta-analysis of 24 selected studies from the period 1951-1979 and found that 47% of the research outcomes showed a positive relationship between religious and mental health variables, whereas a zero relationship was obtained in 30% of cases. When only statistically significant results were included, it was found that 17 % had a positive relationship and 6% had a negative relationship. Two possible explanations were stated. Firstly, the confusing mixture of positive and negative results was due to religion's multi-dimensional nature. Secondly, negative effects of other kinds, which provided unimpressive or ambiguous average effects, were balancing the positive effects of some kinds of religiosity. However, this review demonstrated that there was more support for claims that religion was beneficial to mental health. This view was also shared by Brown (1994) in his concluding remarks to a series of papers on religion, personality, and mental health, saying, "All authors accept that religions can offer preventive and therapeutic resources, most obviously among the poor, homeless, bereaved, and for those who are physically or mentally ill." (p. 193).

Though there is a lack of consensus regarding the impact of religion on mental health, most researchers would agree that religion is not a homogenous, one-dimensional construct. Wilson (1978) had drawn a caution that "religion is not a homogenous whole, individuals who are religious in one respect might not be in another….religion is multidimensional" (p. 442). Later Masters and Bergin (1992) recommended the use of different approaches to provide differentiated levels of investigation in the study of the role of religion in the life of a believer.

Spilda and Werme (1971) pointed out that religion might serve as a means of expressing emotional disturbance, a haven from stress, a source of stress, a means of social acceptance and conformity, or as a means of growth and fulfillment. Clinebell's (1970) analysis of religion as a "sleeping giant" suggested that there was untapped potential in a person's religious faith for the prevention of maladjustment, the fostering of growth and positive mental health.

Identified areas being affected positively and/or negatively by religion (depending on how religion is conceptualized) by Schumaker (1992) are: the mental health of women; sexual expression/adjustment; depression and suicide; anxiety and fear of death; guilt, shame, and self-esteem; rationality; self-actualization, psychological well-being and meaning in life; neuroticism and psychoticism; development in various life stages (e.g., children and the elderly); marital adjustment; crime and delinquency; and alcohol and drug use. There are substantial connections between religion and positive functioning in every area, especially when religion is defined as intrinsic or mature, though there are also detrimental connections. Schumaker's (1992, p.3) elaboration on the positive functions of religion is worth quoting. Religion does:

1. reduce existential anxiety by offering a cognitive structure whereby pacifying explanations and attributions serve to order an otherwise chaotic world;
2. offer a sense of hope, meaning, and purpose along with a resultant sense of emotional well-being;
3. provide a reassuring fatalism that enables one to better withstand suffering and pain;
4. afford solutions to a wide array of situational and emotional conflicts;
5. partially solve the disturbing problem of mortality by way of afterlife beliefs;
6. give people a sense of power and control through association with an omnipotent force;
7. establish self-serving and other-serving moral guidelines, while suppressing self-destructive practices and lifestyles;
8. promote social cohesion;
9. offer a well-focused social identity and satisfies belongingness needs by uniting people around shared understandings; and
10. provide a foundation for cathartic collectively enacted ritual. (p. 3)

A recent review of research on the relation between religion and/or spirituality, and mental health by Koenig (2009), with descriptions of more recent studies in the western countries, found that religious involvement is related to better coping with stress, less depression, suicide, anxiety, and substance abuse.

6.2. Religion as a Protective Factor

Based on a number of empirical studies, many researchers had suggested that religion was a protective factor within an individual, a family, and a community (Hansen, 1992; Koenig, 1998, 2009; Matson & Wells, 1995; Pargament, 1997; Schumaker, 1992). Within an individual, religion could strengthen one's coping skills, self-esteem, and enhance supportive emotional and tangible resources for an individual undergoing major life stress. Within a family, since religion places a primary focus on the sanctity and importance of the family, it helps build up a better marital relationship and facilitate a viable parental support system and that would enhance healthy childhood development. In the community, religion contributes to the needy through congregational outreach programs, which improves the welfare of its community. Some related studies of religion as a protector factor are summarized as follows.

Religion as an individual support and coping

A number of studies have shown that religion is a source of help to individuals who have to cope with life stress. Prayer, scripture, religion ritual, and spiritual support from clergy or church members may facilitate coping with uncontrollable life stressors, such as illness, death, and unemployment. This is done by providing a sense of hope and meaning and facilitating emotional catharsis or processing. Saudia et al.,(1991) studied a group of patients undergoing cardiac surgery, 73% reported that prayer was very helpful to them in preparing for the surgery. Other studies also reported that religion was helpful in coping with their situation such as people with chronic illness and cancer (Raleigh, 1992), or elderly women and men with medical problems (Koenig et al., 1992). Kaplan et al.,(1997) successfully interviewed 53 adult women with HIV. Nearly 40% reported clinically significant levels of depressive symptomatology and anxiety. It was found that prayer and rediscovery of self were their most frequent coping responses.

Sistler and Washington (1999) described an eight-week series of caregiver meetings using the "Serenity Prayer" as a major theme for African-American women caring for a parent with dementia. The prayer is "God grant me the Serenity to accept the things I cannot change, Courage to change the things I can and the Wisdom to know the difference." During the group meetings, the caregivers identified things they could and could not change. It is hypothesized that the Serenity Prayer can provide a quiet mind to the caregivers and assist them to manage their role more effectively. Seven caregivers completed all of the sessions. The interviews consisted of a questionnaire that assessed caregiver well-being, social support, and care receiver status. They were conducted before, after, and six months following the meetings. The results indicated that there was greater self-confidence in the ability to solve difficult situations, improved well-being and happiness, as well as a positive response from the caregivers.

Self-esteem is an important mental health outcome. Krause (1995) examined the relationship between religious coping and self-esteem by interviewing 1,005 elderly people regarding religiosity, education, and self-esteem. It was found that people who relied heavily on religion to cope had very high levels of self-esteem. However, feelings of self-worth appeared to be lowest for those with very little religious commitment compared to those with moderate levels of religious involvement.

Pargament and Brant (1998) summarized the results of 46 studies that examined the relationship between religious orientations and the outcome of critical life events. They explored the basic question of whether people with more religious experience had a more positive or negative outcome of stressful life events than those who were less religious. Religion in these studies was measured as a stable, global, personal disposition - a part of an individual's orienting system. Orienting system was defined as a general way of perceiving and dealing with the world which consisted of values, habits, generalized beliefs, relationships, and personality (Pargament, 1997). These studies targeted people who faced a variety of stressful life events, such as chronic illness, abortion, surgery, and the death of a child, spouse, or loved one. The statistical relationships between religious orientation and outcome for each study were sorted into one of three categories: significantly positive, significantly negative, and non-significant. The results showed that 34% of the statistical relationships between religious orientation and adjustment were significantly positive, whereas about 62% non-significant, and rarely significantly negative. High levels of church involvement, personal religious beliefs, faith, and a more intrinsic religious commitment were also found to relate to beneficial outcome.

Pargament (1997) reviewed 40 studies that examined the statistical relationships between the measures of specific types of religious coping and the outcomes of negative life events. The six different types of religious coping were spiritual coping, congregational coping, religious reframing, religious approaches to agency and control, religious rituals, and combinations of religious coping methods. Most of these studies included more than one measure of religious coping and more than one measure of adjustment. Ignoring the distinctions among the different types of religious coping, it was found that overall 53% of the relationships between religious forms of coping and adjustment were statistically significant. It was suggested that religion was helpful in coping. It may provide comfort, stimulate personal growth, enhance a sense of intimacy with God, and facilitate closeness with others, or offer meaning and purpose in life (Pargament & Park, 1995).

A community-based, longitudinal study starting from 1981on relationships of religious worship attendances and those seeking spiritual comfort with subsequent major depression, anxiety disorders, and suicidal ideation/attempts was conducted. Data from waves 3 taken between 1993 and 1996 with N=1920 and wave 4 collected in 2004 and 2005 with N=1091were used. Results suggest that religious attendance is possibly an independent protective factor against suicide attempts (Rasic et al, 2011).

In short, there were positive evidences supporting that religion could be a protective factor to an individual in response to a life crisis. Different types of religious coping such as prayer, scripture, religious ritual, and support from clergy and church members were found to be effective, especially for those with high level of religious involvements.

Religion as a protective factor in family

Reviews of the empirical literature by Hansen (1992) found a positive relationship between religiousness and marital adjustment. It was suggested that religious norms or values might be especially important for the marital satisfaction of highly religious women. Higher religiosity appeared to explain the fact that individuals in same faith marriages generally report higher adjustment than those in interfaith marriages. Another study by Stinnett (1979) had shown a relationship between strongly religious orientation and strong families. The clear norms provided by religion to family including familial love, solidarity, stability, marital satisfaction, and family priorities might be one of the contributory factors in better marital relationships among more religious parents.

One study on low-income African American parents, found that parents scoring higher on religiousness (behaviors and attitudes) reported greater social support and more favorable parenting practices (Strayhorn, Weidman, & Larson, 1990). The church usually not only emphases on the importance of family, but also provides parenting class, family enrichment programs, and pastoral family counseling to improve member's parenting skills. Furthermore, general emotional support and peer modeling are also likely to contribute to better parenting and the development of protective factors in youth. Thus, religion in the congregational context may facilitate a viable parental support system.

Religion could provide coping resources for children to go through the period of young adulthood. Such resources may include the belief in a loving and protective God, a meaning provided through a religious worldview, emotional release, and a sense of control through prayer and ritual (Shafranske, 1992). One longitudinal study by Werner and Smith (1982) found that the at-risk youth with strong religious faith, who drew support from religious personnel including mentors, ministers, and members of church youth organizations had a more positive life outcome than those lacking these religious resources.

Other studies also show that religion can be a protective factor to family. Mahoney et al.,(2001) conducted a meta-analytic review and conceptual analysis of links between religion, marriage, and parenting. 94 studies published in journals since 1980 were reviewed. Meta-analysis techniques were used to quantify religion-family associations were examined in at least 3 studies. The findings showed that greater religiousness appeared to decrease the risk of divorce and facilitate marital functioning, but the effects were small. Isolated findings also suggested that greater parental religiousness related to more positive parenting and better child adjustment. However, the findings were restricted because of reliance on global or single-item measures of religious and family domain.

Weaver et al.,(2002) conducted a systematic review of quantitative research studies published between 1995 and 1999 in six major marriage and family journals. The findings revealed that 13.2% of them included a measure of religion. This percentage was higher than that found in previous reviews of empirical research in psychological and psychiatric journals, suggesting that marriage and family research journals were more sensitive to the role of religious factors than were those in related disciplines.

Religion as a protective factor in the Community

Some surveys have indicated that the majority of congregational outreach programs are directed toward at-risk families and children in local communities (George et al., 1989; McAdoo & Crawford, 1991). Though such programs vary greatly in content, scope, and costs, they provide social support to parents, educational support to at-risk students, and economic support to poor families. This may have a preventive impact on the community by enhancing family stability and contributing to students' school achievement and attendance.

A study has been conducted to compare the religious and non-religious settings involved in a social and educational outreach effort by providing mentors to at-risk inner city Baltimore youth over a seven-year period (6th-12th grade). The goal of the program was to enhance the social development and school attendance for youth at risk of school dropout and other social problems. Fifth-year evaluation data indicated that students involved with mentors from two sponsoring churches were significantly more likely than students involved with 5 non-religious sponsoring groups (3 companies, 1 college, and 1 fraternal group) to: 1) have a longer term relationship with a mentor; 2) report positive effects from mentoring; and 3) achieve greater attendance, higher school grades, and fewer school withdrawals. These results suggested that religious settings might uniquely contribute to preventive outreach persistence and efficacy, perhaps owing to the religious commitment and congregational support of volunteers (cited in Maton & Wells, 1995).

Other studies also suggested that religion is a protective factor in community in terms of its positive effect on different social issues. Baier and Wright (2001) conducted a meta-analysis on studies published during the period 1967-1998 concerning the effects of religion on crime. They examined60 identified studies concerning the effect of religion on crime and study characteristics. The findings showed that religious beliefs and behaviors exerted a moderate deterrent effect on the individuals' criminal behavior. However, one limitation of the review was that the studies systematically varied in their estimation of the religion-on-crime effect due to differences in conceptual and methodological approaches.

Mason and Windle (2002) conducted a prospective longitudinal study to examine the relationship between religiosity and alcohol use among a sample of middle-adolescent boys and girls. The primary aim of the study was to determine the extent to which religion differentially predicted three outcomes: 1) the decision to use alcohol, 2) the choice among users of how much and how often to drink, and 3) the experience of alcohol-related problems. 840 middle-adolescent boys and girls were recruited to complete measures of religiosity, perceived family social support, peer attachment, school commitment, peer and own alcohol use, and alcohol-related problems. The results using regression analyses revealed that religious salience was associated negatively with later decisions to use alcohol, but the association became non-significant when controlling for peer, family, and school influence. However, religious attendance predicted decreases in the quantity and frequency of alcohol use even in the presence of peer, family, and school variables.

6.3. Religion and Its Effectiveness in Clinical Practices

There are some research findings showing the benefits of religious/spiritual belief and practice in clinical practices. Stark (1971) found that psychiatric patients were far less likely to be religious than so-called normal people. In a study of 100 cases of mentally ill individuals, it was found that they were clearly less religious and less active in a denomination than the matched control subjects who were not mentally ill. Therefore, he challenged the thesis that religion was associated with psychopathology and argued that "psychopathology seems to impede the manifestation of conventional religious beliefs and activities" (p. 175).

In a British epidemiological study, church going and a vital religion were found to be a protective factor from vulnerability to depression (Brown & Prudo, 1981). In a study of 128 black schizophrenic inpatients by Chu and Klein (1985), it was reported that patients were less likely to be re-hospitalized if their families encouraged them to continue religious worshipping while they were in the hospital. On the contrary, patients were more likely to be re-admitted if their families had no religious affiliation. It was suggested that there was a positive correlation between religious worshipping and favorable community outcome. In a 12-year review of all articles appearing in the American Journal of Psychiatry and Archives of General Psychiatry, 72% of the religious commitment variables were beneficial to mental health. Participation in religious services, social support, prayer, and a relationship with God were beneficial in 92% of citations (Larson et al., 1992). Similar findings appeared in a review of the Journal of Family Practice (Craigie et al., 1990).

In a qualitative research project conducted by Sullivan (1993) with 40 respondents who had suffered from serious mental illness but were functioning successfully, it was found that medication, vocational activity, support from friends, and spiritual beliefs were all crucial factors to their success. Additionally, 48% of respondents indicated that their spiritual beliefs helped them solve problems, served as a means of social support, and helped them make sense out of difficult life dilemmas.

Two clinical trials using religious oriented psychotherapy for treating religious patients with either anxiety or depressive disorders showed that patients receiving religious oriented therapy experienced significantly better short-term outcomes (Azhart et al., 1994; Propst et al., 1992). A study by Koenig et al.,(1998) found that among 87 depressed medical inpatients, almost two-thirds of patients indicated that they used religion to “a large extent” to help them cope with their medical problems and other life stressors. Furthermore, it also showed that patients with higher intrinsic religiosity remitted from depression significantly faster than those with lower scores on the intrinsic religiosity scale.

A survey by Fitchett et al.,(1997) on 51 adult psychiatric inpatients about their religious needs and resources, with 50 general patients as a comparison group, found that 80% of the psychiatric patients considered themselves to be a religious or spiritual person (Vs 86% for medical patients), and 88% reported that they had three or more religious or spiritual needs (Vs 76% of medical patients). These needs included “to know God’s presence” (84%), “purpose and meaning in life” (75%), “relief from fear of death” (51%), “prayer” (80%), “receiving sacraments or communion” (39%), “attending religious services” (84%), “care and support from another” (90%), “chaplain visit and pray” (65%) and “visit from a clergy-person” (59%). Furthermore, 68% of the psychiatric patients indicated religion was a source of strength and comfort to them. These findings suggest that many psychiatric patients have spiritual needs which should be taken care of.

Pullen et al.,(1999) investigated relationships between alcohol and drug abuse by adolescents and the frequency of religious service attendance in the south-east United States. Data collected from surveys of 217 adolescents, age 12-19 years, were analyzed. The adolescents included participants from both clinical and non-clinical settings. Results from both groups showed that, as attendance of religious services increased, alcohol and drug abuse decreased. The study is consistent with many previous studies that religiosity does influence an adolescent’s alcohol and drug abuse. Thus, they support the possibility of including spiritual/religious interventions in any alcohol and/or drug treatment program.

Tepper et al.,(2001) conducted a survey on 13 Los Angeles County mental health facilities to examine the prevalence of religious coping among individuals with persistent mental illness. Four hundred and six patients were recruited. A questionnaire consisted of the Religious Coping Index, the Symptom Checklist 90-R (SCL-90), the Global Assessment of Functioning, and a 48 item demographic questionnaire was used. The findings showed that more than 80% of the participants used religious beliefs or activities to cope with daily difficulties or frustrations. Prayer was the most frequently used coping strategy. The amount of time that participants devoted to religious coping was negatively related to reported levels of frustration and scores on the SCL-90 symptom subscales. The study concluded that religion might serve as a pervasive and potentially effective method of coping for individuals with mental illness, and it is recommended to have religion integrated into psychiatric and psychological practice.

In a survey study conducted by Russinova et al (2002) regarding the types of alternative healthcare practices used by 157 adults with severe mental illness, it was found that the most common beneficial alternative health practice was religious or spiritual activities.

In a systematic review of the effects of religion-accommodative psychotherapy for depression and anxiety, results from the 11 studies reviewed indicate that psychotherapy integrating religion is at least as effective for treating depression and anxiety as other forms of non-religious psychotherapy. When compared with less stringent control groups, such as supportive psychotherapy, religion-accommodative therapy may be more effective (Paukert et al., 2011).

To sum up, as suggested by Kelly (1995), recent data “do not permit drawing a causal link between religiousness and good emotional health, nonetheless some evidence suggests that in certain cases clients’ spirituality and religiousness offer a set of personal characteristics and dynamics that may be useful in the clients’ development and problem solving” (p. 83). As caring professionals, we have to be aware and be sensitive to our clients’ divergent spiritual/religious beliefs and practices. We need to be prepared not only to work with those unhealthy religious beliefs and practices that may affect our clients’ mental health but also to strengthen those positive elements of the clients’ religiousness that could enhance their rehabilitation process.

6.4. Existing Psychiatric Rehabilitation Programs with Explicit Religious Elements

Despite the paucity of psychiatric rehabilitation programs with explicit religious or spiritual elements, there are still some representative programs existing both locally and overseas. With regard to overseas programs, the Alcoholics Anonymous, Emotional Anonymous, and GROW will be discussed.

As suggested by Polich, Armor, and Braiker (1981), the single most effective intervention for alcoholism is Alcoholics Anonymous (AA) which facilitates fundamental changes in the alcoholic's belief system, provides an unambiguous conception of the illness that is meaningful to the client, and gives a sense of hope in the possibility of recovery. It is consistent with the findings of a longitudinal study by Vaillant (1983) on alcoholism. One of the conditions found directly to precede stable recovery from alcoholism was increased involvement in religion or some analogous spiritual or ideological experience. Such an experience typically helped the alcoholic replace feelings of defeat, worthlessness, helplessness, and guilt with renewed hope, self-esteem, and a powerful new belief system that enabled him to swear off his old maladaptive life-style for a new one. Levine and Perkins (1987) also suggested that the fellowship and support provided by other AA members, both during the regular meetings and when needed at other times and places, were a powerful reinforcer in the life of the isolated alcoholic and induced strong tendencies to affiliate and identify.

The entire program of AA is a tripartite as suggested by Talbott (1990) including physical, emotional, and spiritual aspects. The spiritual aspect, which states that a power outside of the individual, a force greater than the individual, is necessary for their recovery, and is a critical component of the success of AA. The central part to the philosophy of AA is the concept of Divine intervention by a Higher Power, which is apparent in six of its 12-steps program reflecting the origins of AA in an English Protestant sect called the Oxford Group. They are listed as follows (cited in Ellis and Schoenfeld, 1990).

2. Came to believe that a Power greater than ourselves could restore us to sanity.
3. Made a decision to turn our will and our lives over to the care of God as we understood Him.
5. Admitted to God, to ourselves, and to another human being the

exact nature of our wrongs.

6. Were entirely ready to have God remove all these defects of character.
7. Humbly asked Him to remove our shortcomings.
11. Sought through prayer and meditation to improve our conscious contact with God as we understood Him, praying only for knowledge of His will for us and the power to carry that out.

An AA group consists of meetings, which all members are encouraged to attend. The frequency varies considerably according to the individual group. Members may take years to complete the steps, and will be understood and accepted if they have failed. The meeting is usually divided into several parts. It customarily begins with a reading of the "Prayer of Serenity". Then different members might read some basic materials, such as the 12-steps and then an experienced member delivers a speech. The most important part of the meeting follows, which is when the members could freely share their positive experiences. Then the meeting concludes with announcements, coffee, and general socializing (Katz, 1993).

The AA group was first started in 1935 and was later widely accepted as a self-help organization for alcoholics. In mid-1970s, three new groups that emphasized behavior modification through reliance on self rather than a higher power were formed. They were Rational Recovery (RR), Save Our Selves/Secular Organization for Sobriety (SOS), and Women for Sobriety (WFS). However, there are no reliable studies comparing these groups with AA (Uva, 1991). On the other hand, many studies had supported the efficacy of religiously oriented 12-steps programs (Alford et al., 1991; Brown & Peterson, 1991; Carroll, 1993). Alford et al.,(1991) evaluated the outcomes of 12-step interventions in adolescent inpatients. They found that 75% of adolescents who completed the 12 step-oriented treatments were abstinent at the end of treatment, as compared to only 35% of non-completers. In addition, regardless of completion of the program, subjects who attended AA less often were less likely to be abstinent than those inpatients attending meetings more frequently. Brown and Peterson (1991) examined the use of spiritual practices endorsed by 12-step programs among 35 successfully recovering alcoholics. These practices included practicing meditation/quiet time/relaxing (100%), engaging in the practice of prayer (100%), and regular reading of spiritual literature or personal growth books (91%). It was also discovered that frequent use of these spiritual practices significantly predicted successful recovery among alcoholics. Carroll (1993) had also reported that prayer and meditation (step 11), along with regular AA attendance, were positively associated with the length of sobriety and purpose in life of AA members.

Emotions Anonymous (EA) was started in Minnesota in 1971, and adopted AA's "Twelve Steps" and "Twelve Traditions". It is open to anyone who wants to achieve emotional well-being. EA members' goals are serenity and peace of mind. EA views emotional ill health as a chronic and progressive physical, mental, and spiritual illness. EA members come to believe that there is a higher power and become willing to accept help. In EA, surrender to a higher power does not mean complete passivity. Instead, such surrender reflects an acceptance of reality as it exists and a cessation of efforts to "play God".

Each EA group meets once a week and members can and do attend more than one group each week. During the group meeting, members take turns reading from the group's literature and share their experiences following the 12 step principles. The meeting ends with a closing statement and also a prayer. However, a group may change this format by discussing a topic other than one of the 12-Steps and may allow more interaction during the discussion. A study by Kurtz and Chambon (1987) suggests that EA is a viable resource for a large percentage of those who attend EA meetings. It has been well received in most large metropolitan areas, as well as in some smaller communities, for those who are prone to chronic worry, tension, and are compulsive with ineffective efforts at control.

GROW was founded in Sydney in 1957 by a Roman Catholic priest and other anonymous members with mental illness. GROW has its root in AA and changes the area of concern to rehabilitation problems of former psychiatric patients. The philosophy of the GROW program consists of three key elements. The first is the "Twelve Stages of Decline", which basically describes how one moves from using neurotic defense to harboring chronic psychotic symptoms. The second is the "will to get well", which emphasizes the essential motive for one to reverse the process of decline back to maturity. The third element is the "twelve steps of personal growth", which illustrate the process from maladjustment to maturity. Among the latter, in the third step "we surrender to the healing power of God", shows the spiritual dimension of the intervention by surrendering to the healing power of God in response to one's self-centeredness. In the eighth step "we learn to think by reason rather than by feelings and imagination" and in the ninth step "we train our wills to govern our feelings" demonstrates the emphasis of rationality in controlling one's life.

GROW's objective is to assist members in attaining mental, social, and spiritual maturity. Help comes to members through self-activation, mutual help, and surrender to God. Group intervention is the basic intervention for all members to achieve maturity. Each group session lasts for about two hours and is divided into two major parts. In the first part, members are required to recite certain messages from the "Grow Wisdom", which are actually compiled from papers presented by members to the GROW meeting leaders. These reading materials have been seen to be helpful to a significant number of members. The second part is for group interaction, when members freely share their feelings and urgent problems, so that they can help one another to remove the problems and barricades from the outer world. GROW has over 400 groups throughout Australia and is even spreading to other countries such as the U.K. and the U.S.A. (Yip, 1992).

Beyond these representative rehabilitation programs, there are also some small studies concerning the spiritual dimension of the program in recent literature. Muffler et al.,(1995), in examining four religious based programs for substance dependence, found that religious based programs had a better outcome than secular interventions. Furthermore, it was found that treatment attendance was negatively related to cocaine use post-treatment and cocaine and marijuana use at 6-month follow-up. In addition, patients who attended spiritually based programs wcrc much more likely to report abstinence from opioids one year after the program. In examining a group of 12 clients who participated in a weekly spiritual issues group of a psychiatric day treatment program, O'Rourke (1997) found that the spiritual issues group functioned as a transitional space for clients between communities of support. Furthermore, the group provided members with opportunities for corrective religious and emotional experiences. In the same vein, Kehoe (1999) with 18 years' experience in conducting group therapy focusing on religious issues with chronic psychiatric patients, advocated a group focused on religious issues could provide clients with valuable therapeutic experiences in tolerance, acceptance of other's views, and thoughtful examination of belief systems, as well as opportunities to apply spirituality and values to life questions. Furthermore, concerns that the discussion of religious and spiritual material would foster patients' delusion ideation or strengthen their defenses and be counter-productive to treatment have not been supported.

Locally, there are several drug rehabilitation programs based on Christian belief. Some are highlighted for discussion. St. Stephen's Society, which was established locally by a missionary, Jackie Pullinger in 1966, was one of the largest associations using a religious approach in drug rehabilitation in Hong

Kong (Woo, 1983). In the St. Stephen's Society program, a clear message is given that only Jesus can make one change and with the help from God, chronic drug abusers could be changed into non-drug abusing religious individuals (St. Stephen's Society, 1997). Prayers, individual counseling by ex-drug abusers, Bible readings, worship, religious community, and ultimately baptism are therapeutic measures to free one from the control of drugs to become a new born Christian.

Wu Oi Christian Center was established in 1973 with a religious treatment and rehabilitation program developed to help drug dependent individuals, former prisoners, and problem youths to abstain from heroin addiction. The program consisted of a year-long treatment course and a six-month follow up. It emphasized on the belief of Christian faith and the mutual support from peers especially from those who had successfully overcome the addiction. During the residential treatment course, the center adopted a simple and disciplined lifestyle in a Christian therapeutic community for drug detoxification and rehabilitation (Action Committee Against Narcotics, 2002, p. 84).

The Christian New Being Fellowship was established in 1989. It provided a residential treatment and rehabilitation program with Christian beliefs for youngsters who abused drugs, including psychological substances. The program consisted of individual and group counseling, general education studies, life skills, disciplinary and vocational training, as well as Bible studies (Action Committee Against Narcotics, 2002, p. 80).

Christian Oi Hip Fellowship, the target organization for investigation in this book, is the leading organization of SHGs for former psychiatric patients in Hong Kong. The philosophy of the organization is to provide holistic care to former psychiatric patients, with great emphasis on the spiritual dimension. The details of the organization and its programs will be discussed thoroughly later in this book.

Chapter 7

Self Help Group (SHG)/Mutual Aid Group in Psychiatric Rehabilitation

The group approach in treatment has been widely applied in its many different forms to mental health problems over several decades in western countries (Bednur & Kaul, 1978). Its significant role in the community care of the mentally ill and their families has also been well recognized (Salem, et al., 1988). In the second half of the twentieth century, SHGs have had a dynamic, spectacular rise (Katz, 1993). In this section, the historical development, and the roles and functions of the SHG will be discussed. A comprehensive review of its development in psychiatric rehabilitation in Hong Kong is highlighted. The terms self-help and mutual aid have been used interchangeably and are synonymous in this book. Mutual aid is also used because SHGs emphasize both self-help and mutual aid.

7.1. Historical Development of SHGs

Self-help is not a new phenomenon and has deep historical roots. Kropotkin (1955) argued that cooperation was a basic survival mechanism for human beings. He provided many examples throughout history of spontaneously developed cooperative enterprises and associations for purposes of greater mutual protection and productivity. In medieval guilds, for example, members banded together to regulate their trade. Together the members of a guild constituted a brotherhood, and each was responsible not only for maintaining the standards of the trade but also for providing fraternal benefits to the membership, such as aid in the event of illness, to widows and orphans, and celebrations of births and marriages.

Well into the twentieth century, self-help found newer expressions. In the United States, unions and self-help associations were seen growing in the earlier part of the century. From the 1930s till the 1950s, the philosophy of "a problem shared is a problem eased" was in groups such as AA, Recidivists Anonymous, and Gamblers Anonymous. From then onwards till the 1970s, self-help was said to be politicized, associated with the civil rights movement, the women's movement, consumer groups, and the like. More recently, service-oriented self-help groups and activities have been prominent (Pancoast, Parker, & Froland, 1987).

These different manifestations of self-help in the United States have demonstrated its responsiveness to "the demands of the times", which Pancoast et al.,(1987) specifies as the context within which self-help, in its new forms, becomes an important force. According to Pancoast et al.,(1987), this is a response to economic, political, social, democratic, and social welfare demands.

Nowadays, different models of SHGs or organizations have developed, reflecting their adaptive nature to meet the demand of the times. The emergence of SHGs could be attributed to strong professionalization, service fragmentation, de-personalization and de-humanization of institutions, social alienation, loss of sense of control and choices, raised sense of self-determination, and self-advocacy (Chan et al., 1992; Gartner & Riessman, 1982; Levine & Perkins, 1987). This concept is also shared with the community care approach of community development (Wong, 1992; Wong, 1994). In fact, the development of SHGs is considered as one part of the community-care approach (Wong & Chan, 1994).

7.2. Definition of SHG

There are different definitions of self-help groups; some are more elaborative while others are precise. However, they are not in conflict but complement each other to provide a more comprehensive picture of the SHG. Some commonly used definitions are discussed as follows:

SHG is referred to as "voluntary associations among individuals who share a common need or problem, and who seek to use the group as a means of dealing with that need or problem" (Gartner & Reissman, 1977).

"SHGs are characterized by common experience, mutual help and support, sharing of practical skills in coping, collective will power and belief, importance of information, and constructive action toward shared goals" (Robinson & Henry, 1977, p. 29).

"SHGs are small group structures for mutual aid in the accomplishment of a specific purpose. They are usually formed by peers who have come together for mutual assistance in satisfying a common need, overcoming a common handicap or life-disrupting problem, and bringing about desired social and /or personal change" (Katz & Bender, 1976, p. 9).

"SHGs consist of people who share common conditions, experiences, or problematic situations and mutually seek to assist one another to enhance their coping capacities related to their common factors. The help these groups provide is available without charge and is based on the experiences of members rather than professional expertise. Largely self-governing and self-regulating, self-help groups generally have effective communication networks among members that, in addition to regular group meetings, provide opportunities for both telephone and face-to-face contacts" (Hepworth & Larsen, 1986, p. 549).

A more recent definition developed by Rootes and Aanes (1992) is based on seven criteria:

1) A self-help group is supportive and educational.
2) Its leadership comes from within the group.
3) The group addresses a single major life-disrupting event.
4) Group members participate voluntarily.
5) The group has no monetary interests or profit orientation.
6) The primary purpose of group membership is individual personal growth.
7) Membership is anonymous and confidential since members mostly dislike to have their identity disclosed especially if their problems are sources of stigma such as mental illness, drug addiction etc.

Every definition has shed light in the understanding of the characteristics SHGs. Riessman (1987) has made a very good summary of the distinctive characteristics of SHGs and is illustrated as follows:

- "a noncompetitive, cooperative orientation;
- an anti-elite, anti-bureaucratic focus;
- an emphasis on the indigenous people who have the problem and know a lot about it from the inside, from experiencing it;
- an attitude of do what you can, one day at a time; you can't solve everything at once;
- a shared, often revolving leadership;
- an attitude of being helped through helping (the helper-therapy principle);
- an understanding that helping is not a commodity to be bought and sold;
- a strong optimism regarding the ability to change;
- an understanding that although small may not necessarily be beautiful, it is the place to begin and the unit to build on;
- a critical stance toward professionalism, which is often seen as pretentious, purist, distant, and mystifying; self-helpers like simplicity and informality;
- an emphasis on the consumer;
- an understanding that helping is at the center - knowing how to receive help, give help, and help yourself;
- an emphasis on empowerment" (p. ix-x).

Since many practitioners have difficulty distinguishing among self-help, support, or psychotherapy groups, Rootes & Aanes (1992) differentiate SHGs from support groups in that the latter are not focused on personal growth. Support groups generally deal with an external crisis, and their purpose is to assist members emotionally and educationally until the crisis is past. Powell (1990) suggests that the public tends to use 'support group' as a generic term to refer to professionally controlled groups and self-help/mutual aid groups to those that are primarily owned by consumers.

As suggested by Corey (1990), SHGs and therapy groups have some common denominators in that both encourage and support, stress the value of affiliation, and aim for behavioral change. Despite these commonalties between self-help and therapy groups, there are some critical differences. Unlike SHGs, which have their central issue as a single topic, therapy groups have more global goals such as improving general mental health or one's interpersonal functioning. Therapy groups also emphasize professional leadership and serve as a social microcosm. However, these differences are not so distinctive since some SHGs also possess these functions.

A more precise distinction between self-help, support, and psychotherapy groups is made by Kurtz (1997) who proposed that a major difference between self-help and support is that the former aims at effecting change. While the difference between self-help and a psychotherapy group is that a professional therapist conducts the latter. In using a continuum, Schopler and Galinsky (1995) place self-help on one-end and psychotherapy groups on the other, with support groups in between and potentially overlapping on either end.

For simplicity of understanding, the definition by Katz and Bender (1976) is adopted in this book.

7.3. Self Help Group and Social Work

Social welfare has been broadly defined by the National Association of Social Workers as "The full range of organized activities of voluntary and governmental agencies that seek to prevent, alleviate, or contribute to the solution of recognized social problems, or to improve the well-being of individuals, groups, or communities. Such activities use a wide variety of professional personnel such as physicians, nurses, lawyers, educators, engineers, ministers, and social workers." (Pumphrey, 1977, p. 1446). While suggested by Doloff and Feldstein (1980), social work is the major professional group in the social welfare arena for the delivery of social welfare services. Historically, professional social workers have been using both individual casework and group work as social treatment for their clients. However, an issue is raised that there is a relative neglect of group work in terms of the SHG being used by social workers. Adams (1990) suggested several possible reasons. Firstly, some social workers undervalue the activities of self-help. Secondly, the conceptual confusion inhibits social work involvement in self-help and finally, empowerment through self-help is under-developed. Wasserman and Danforth (1988) suggested that some social workers are prone to high values which can be immediately applicable to working with individuals and families. Furthermore, clinical social workers are more primarily interested in individual treatments, which are drawn from theories of psychotherapy. On the other hand, the very naturalness of the self-help "method" raises doubt in professionals.

Despite the lack of attention to SHGs, some professional social workers have a very positive attitude towards the SHG. Lieberman and Borman (1979) found that many professional social workers had been involved at early phases of group organization. A few professionals had actively participated in starting SHGs. An example was Leonard Lieber, a social worker, who was one of the founders of Parents Anonymous, an SHG for parents of abused children (Katz, 1993).

Wasserman and Danforth (1988) advocated that social work is the sole discipline with the historical tradition and the appropriate organization of services to create, maintain and strengthen the support systems for people. Moreover, the formation of support groups in the form of SHGs ought to be a part of every social work agency. They further recommended that both social casework and social group work are important. Some clients need only individual casework while others require only an SHG. However, some can benefit from a combination of the two. Comstock and Mohamoud (1990) supported that there are benefits for both the members and professionals in the professionally-facilitated SHG. Social workers can benefit from the SHG both in professional knowledge and personal growth. A study by Wituk et al.,(2000) using telephone interviews of 253 SHG representatives in Kansas showed that many SHGs have shared leadership, receive assistance from professional social workers, and guidance from national and local organizations.

Recently, there are an increasing number of articles in social work literature on the use of support groups in practice. Using the words "mutual aid group", or "SHG" or "group work" in Social Work Abstract for searching, there are 672 articles during the years 1980 to 1990, and 727 articles during 1991 till 2004, found respectively. Nearly every field of social work has introduced professionally-initiated groups, such as school social work, family and children's' services, healthcare services etc.

7.4. Types of SHGs

Since there are different varieties of SHGs, many authorities have attempted to make their descriptions as classifications of SHGs. Some representative typologies are described as follows.

Based on purpose and composition, Levy (1976) proposes a four-folded classification. Type I groups emphasize conduct re-organization or behavioral control. "Alcoholics Anonymous", "Take Off Pounds Sensibly", and "Parents Anonymous" are among groups representative of this type. Type II groups are those with members sharing a predicament which entails a degree of stress.

Their aim is not to change the situation but to reduce stress. Examples include, "Parents Without Partners" and "Make Today Count". Type III groups are survival-oriented with members that society has discriminated against or labeled deviant. The groups' aims include both mutual support and the raising of consciousness to enhance self-esteem, with publicity and political activity aimed at societal acceptance and the elimination of discrimination. Black pride and homosexual groups would fall in this category. Members of the Type IV groups share goals of personal growth, self-actualization, and enhanced effectiveness in life. There is no central, shared concern but members bring their problems to such a group in the belief that together members can help each other to better lives. A sensitivity group is an example of such a group. Though Levy's description could provide a useful way to classify the different nature of groups, it is insufficient to cover the variety of groups that have sufficient characteristics in common, to be treated as related phenomenon.

Levine and Perkins (1987) provide a more detailed analysis of the five types of SHGs. The first type involves people whose state or condition leads to some disqualification from being "normal". Members of these groups exhibit behavior or have characteristics that subject them to social isolation, stigmatization, scorn, pity, or social punishment. Examples are alcoholics, individuals with diagnoses of mental illness, ex-convicts, gamblers, drug addicts, homosexuals and those with physical characteristics or illnesses, such as dwarfs and the physically handicapped.

The second type of SHG is made up of those related to people with stigmatizing conditions, who themselves may be subject to some secondary stigma or who suffer consequences because of the problems presented by the person related to them. Examples are spouses and children of alcoholics, gamblers, and the mentally ill.

A third type of group includes people with common problems that may not be stigmatizing but that do tend to be socially isolating. Public resources may be inadequate, and others who do not have the problem may not understand the individual's or the family's situation. Examples are groups for widows, groups for single parents, etc.

A fourth type is a group organized along ethnic, religious, or racial lines for mutual assistance. These include fraternal organizations that provide education, recreation, cultural preservation, insurance, prepaid medical care, and similar services.

A fifth type is organized along quasi-political lines for the preservation of specific interests. These include taxpayers' groups seeking to limit taxation, civic organizations designed to preserve the character of neighborhoods, and organizations concerned with community development.

Though Levine's classification considers a wider perspective, it is difficult to apply because there are rarely pure forms of any one type of group, and most groups fit into more than one category.

Based on resource dependence and authority to make decisions, Schubert and Borkman (1991) identified the five types of SHGs according to their dependence on a larger organization.

1. Unaffiliated groups - independent local group with no relationship of an outside source of leadership, funding or policy.
2. Federated groups - groups relating to a larger association but have complete autonomy.
3. Affiliated groups - groups subordinating to higher levels of their own organization.
4. Managed groups - groups monitored and controlled by professionals and under the control of a non-self-help organization.
5. Hybrid groups - groups combining features of affiliated and managed groups. Both peer helpers and professionals cooperate to resolve member difficulties.

The self-help organization of this book, the "Christian Oi Hip Fellowship", is of the first type of SHG as classified by Levine and Perkins (1987), as the Fellowship is made up of former psychiatric patients with stigmatizing conditions. Furthermore, the typology used by Schubert and Borkman (1991) as hybrid groups, is also valid since most mental health professionals organize the Fellowship with a partnership of peer helpers. The structure of the Fellowship will be described in detail in a later section.

7.5. Growth of the SHG

SHGs have been defined earlier as structures designed for the accomplishment of a specific purpose. Intervention with SHGs is not only influenced by the unique character of the groups, but also their stages of developmental growth. Katz (1970) has delineated five stages in the growth of SHGs. They are:

Stage 1: Origin - The period at which the ideal of the group is formulated and preliminary discussions are held among interested individuals.

Stage 2: Informal Organization - The stage at which a group of individuals with a common problem have agreed to meet occasionally on an informal basis to discuss problems and needs.

Stage 3: Emergence of Leadership - A formal leader may be designated at this stage. This may be differentiated from earlier stages in which informal leaders guided the group.

Stage 4: Beginning of Formal Organization - In this stage, the group becomes solidified and developed into a point at which its structure becomes formalized. It elects officers, adopts by laws, follows procedural rules and may adopt a logo, organizational stationery and other materials.

Stage 5: Beginning of Professionalization - In this stage, the formal organization has grown to a point where it may start to hire professionals with expertise in the problem areas.

These identified stages of development are useful as a reference to SHGs' developmental and maintenance processes. However, not all SHGs pass through all these stages and some may never reach stage 5 because of resistance to bureaucratic structure. Furthermore, there may be certain variations in each stage, for example, in the original stage the group may be initiated by either professionals or people with same needs, or in a partnership model like the one of the Fellowship, which is the subject of study in this book.

7.6. Roles of the Healthcare Professionals in SHGs

There are few SHGs that are purely started and developed by the members themselves. On the other hand, many of them have been initiated and supported by professionals behind the scenes. It has been suggested professionals can play a variety of roles in working with SHGs. Those roles include (Smith, 1996; Toseland & Hacker, 1982):

1) identifying and encouraging motivated, energetic, and talented patients or the patients' family members to get involved in forming the groups,

2) providing material support to maintain SHGs,
3) serving as a linkage by connecting traditional services, clients, and SHGs to one another,
4) serving as a consultant to a SHG,
5) serving as educational speakers at group meetings,
6) referring patients as part of treatment protocols.

SHGs are built on peer education and leadership; some groups have a strong anti-professional profile, while others invite professional help (Maton, 1988; Stewart, 1990). Since autonomy and empowerment are important characteristics of an SHG, some members might dislike the involvement of professionals who would dominate the group. Some previous studies suggested that when professionals began a group, they were likely to remain in control of it whether they wanted to be or not (Cherniss & Cherniss, 1987; Yoak & Chesler, 1985). On the other hand, some SHGs might fear that they are not capable of managing themselves and would lose their direction during the group's development, so they have invited professionals of various degrees for help, ranging from consultation to actually participating in their groups as facilitators. A nationwide survey by Emerick (1990) on SHGs for individuals with mental illness placed organizations into three categories:

a) “partnership groups” that allowed professionals to participate in the leadership;
b) “supportive groups” that accepted professionals in auxiliary roles; and
c) “separatist groups” that rejected professionals within their membership in any capacity. It was found that 62% of the groups fell into the supportive category. 21% were “partnership groups” and 16% were “separatist groups”.

It seems there is a general tendency that professional interaction with SHGs is desirable and professionals should support and not replace informal mutual-help efforts. Yoak and Chesler’s (1985) study showed that groups with shared leadership were the largest, most long-lived, and most active. A follow-up study of those groups 10 years later indicated the same pattern (Chesler & Chesney, 1995). However, as suggested by Ma (1992), some mental health professionals were still skeptical about SHGs, which was one of the factors affecting its development. A study by Mok (1997) showed that nurses seldom referred patients to SHGs because of lack of information about SHGs and lack of preparation for the appropriate roles.

Mallory (1984) considered some specific issues that professionals would need to address. Most critically, the professional role must change as the SHG develops. Initially, the professionals can be a generator, a catalyst, or an organizer of the group, and there are multiple models that professionals play in these roles. As the group develops, the professionals must shift their responsibilities so that the group would increasingly develop autonomy, independence, and its own power. Thus, the professionals must become disengaged from their more energetic initial role.

7.7. The Religious SHGs

Many SHGs are formed with the aim to meet the needs of different groups of clients. Some of these SHGs are with an explicit religious or spiritual element, which is the essential component to bring about the recovery of group members. The most representative overseas religious SHGs are the AA, EA, and GROW described in the previous section. As suggested by Talbott (1990), the entire program of AA includes the physical, emotional, and spiritual aspects. The spiritual aspect emphasizes the Divine intervention by a Higher Power for the recovery from alcoholism. Many studies support the efficacy of the religiously oriented 12-steps AA program (Alford et al., 1991; Brown & Peterson, 1991; Carroll, 1993).

EA is another religious SHG which helps members achieve emotional well-being. EA members come to believe that there is a Higher Power and become willing to accept help. It is suggested that EA is a viable resource for a large percentage of those who attend their meetings (Kurtz & Chambon, 1987). With its root in AA, GROW was founded in Sydney for the rehabilitation of former psychiatric patients. One of the interventions of this religious SHG is to surrender to the healing power of God in response to one's centeredness. GROW is found to be effective and has over 400 groups throughout Australia and even spreading to other countries such as the UK and the U S A. (Yip, 1992).

Besides these representative religious SHGs, there are also some recent studies showing the effectiveness of other overseas religious or spiritual SHGs (Kehoe, 1999; Muffler et al., 1995; O'Rourke, 1997). In Hong Kong, there are also some religious SHGs for rehabilitation. Most of them are formed for drug rehabilitation (Action Committee Against Narcotics, 2002). No religious SHG is found for the rehabilitation of former psychiatric patients so far except the

Fellowship, the target organization for this study. However, no formal study is conducted to evaluate the effectiveness of this religious SHG.

7.8. The Effectiveness of SHGs

There has been advocacy about the benefits and advantages offered by the SHG since its development. Caplan (1974) advocated that participation in an SHG reduced the vulnerability and/or acute stress affecting a person at risk. Like any significant social-support system, an SHG can profitably be compared with the model of an ideal family. Social support is an enduring set of relationships with one or more significant others or groups, which help to deal with life stresses or provide special assistance in dealing with particular long-term burdens or stressful situations.

Riessman (1976), and later with Gartner (1982), proposed that the power of SHGs derived from their combining a number of very important properties: the helper-therapy principle, group reinforcement, continuous intervention, an ideological perspective, and the implicit demand that the individual would do something for himself. They enable their members to feel and use their strengths and power to exert control over their own lives. The effectiveness and some potential problems of SHGs as postulated by some researchers are discussed in the following paragraphs.

Pilisuk and Minkler (1985) postulated the mutual-help revolution contributed not only to the combating of loneliness and the building of community, but also to the prevention of illness and recovery from disease. For those who become ill, social support also may help predict the likelihood of recovery, the amount of medication required, and the patient‘s ability to adhere to a therapeutic regimen of diet, medication, or exercise.

The self-help ethos has been considered as the most important force in maintaining the self-help movement. Riessman and Gartner (1987) suggested the strength of the self-help movement derived from its spirit, the self-help ethos. The self-help ethos is a constellation of norms and sentiments. It is an ideal type of construction and no one SHG possesses all the dimensions of the self-help ethos. The five major dimensions of self-help ethos are: (i) anti-big; (ii) reaffirmation of traditions; (iii) empowerment and participation; (iv) new-age psychology; and (v) democratization. These dimensions are briefly described as follows.

(i) *Anti-big (e.g., anti-bureaucratic)*
It reflects a response to bureaucracy and hierarchy in modern society. It emphasizes face-to face relations. Members of common problems are encouraged to articulate their experiences with professionals to reduce professional distance. Authority and power are distributed in a flattened hierarchy. Bureaucracy is replaced by simple small groups and social networks.

(ii) *Reaffirmation of traditions (e.g., community, neighbor-hood, belonging)*
This is a cry against the breakdown of norms and positive traditions such as intimate human relationships, mutual support, and cooperation, and sense of belonging which are compatible with the Chinese traditions. Important components of social networks such as family, neighborhood, relatives, friends, and volunteers are crucial components to translate these values into practice.

(iii) *Empowerment (e.g., self-determination)*
The sense of having control over one's life, and expanding the consumer's role in human services is facilitated through empowerment and participation. Member participation and determination are based on the belief that members are the only ones who understand their situations the most. Through the process of empowerment, the problem-solving ability is improved with enhancement in self-image and confidence.

(iv) *New Age Psychology (e.g., de-isolation, self-acceptance)*
De-isolation and self-actualization are two core concepts. Through the process of self-acceptance and normalization, feelings such as isolation and alienation are minimized. This theme represents a significant breakthrough releasing enormous energy and re-framing self-images and self-esteem.

(v) *Democratization of everyday life (e.g., anti-elite, anti-expert)*
Democratic theme extends from a personal level to a group level. At the personal level, the accent is on the operation of values including acceptance of difference and openness. At the group level, the theme emphasizes the advocacy of citizen rights and participation. Antagonistic

to the emphasis on the experiential wisdom, elitism, and expertise are underplayed in this theme.

Levine and Perkins (1987) identified six aspects of self-help that serve its members' interests. SHGs 1) promote the psychological sense of community; 2) provide an ideology that serves as a philosophical antidote; 3) provide an opportunity for confession, catharsis, and mutual criticism; 4) provide role models; 5) teach effective coping strategies for day-to-day problems; and 6) provide a network of social relationships.

Rutchick (1990) presented an outline of the therapeutic forces available in small groups as follows:

(i) Universalization - the shared understanding that one's experiences and feelings are not unique often diminishes feelings of isolation and alienation.

(ii) Models for identification - both the success and failure of others provide a yardstick for measuring one's own performance.

(iii) Sharing of information - inclusion of both didactic instruction from experts, as well as shared experiences and knowledge among members facilitates mastery.

(iv) Emotional catharsis - shared painful or "unacceptable" experiences and feelings that are accepted by others can be liberating and growth producing.

(v) Reality testing - feedback from others, as well as the displaced "confrontation" provided by observing how others cope, can provide an accurate perception of one's strengths and liabilities.

(vi) Peer support - the provision of advice and understanding to others helps to enhance self-esteem by permitting an individual to be in a giving, as well as receiving /dependent role.

(vii) Hope - the opportunity to see the progress of others in a similar situation permits comparisons and opens avenues of optimism.

(viii) Practice in communication - group norms and support for communicating without condemning and for listening can improve the quality of interpersonal interaction.

Belton (1994) mentioned that most of the SHGs are based on small group theory. According to Shulman and Gitterman (1994), there are a number of mutual processes that can be identified when one watches an effective small group in action. These processes include: sharing data; the dialectical process;

entering taboo areas; the "all in the same boat" phenomenon; mutual support; mutual demand; individual problem-solving; rehearsal; and the strength in numbers phenomenon.

Despite a long list of theoretical views about the effectiveness of SHGs as mentioned above, potential problems of the SHG are also raised by several writers. Henry and Robinson (1978) pointed to the possibility that there might be potential harm when a person who was actually in need of other professional services such as individual therapy was inappropriately referred to an SHG. For example, severe depression may need intervention from a psychiatrist who would prescribe drug treatment, which could reasonably address the client's problem. However, Lieberman (1990) found that most individuals who participate in SHGs ordinarily receive a variety of services.

As a president of a self-help organization for Anorexia Nervosa and Associated Disorders, Rubel (1984) raised several potential problems of the SHG, which should require precaution. Firstly, since the SHG emphasizes on personal responsibility, if the individual fails to change in the SHG, there is a risk that these individuals will be blamed and stigmatized, which would lead to a form of victim-blaming. In fact, many possible causes such as the group leadership skills, the make-up of the group membership, and failure of the medical intervention will all cause the ineffectiveness of the group treatment. On the other hand, some individuals may go into a form of escapism since many SHGs teach their members to rely on a "higher power" to help them but prematurely and not constructively. The members become more and more dependent on an external authority without exploring and fully utilizing their own ability. Thirdly, some members of the group that have received or are receiving professional therapy, may play the role of junior therapist and make inappropriate suggestions during group sessions, which may damage the mutuality in the group. The same problem may arise if in a professional-supported group, the professional attempts to dominate the group, which would also damage the mutually supportive effort of the SHG. As mentioned by Gartner and Riessman (1977), some members might perceive that an SHG is the last resort they could turn to for their problems. If they drop out of the group because of whatever reason, they may experience severe depression, feelings of failure and inadequacy, and painfully negative self-esteem. The last problem is that SHGs seldom keep records or any kind of systematic evaluation of their activities. This would lead to great difficulties in determining accountability and effectiveness.

Chesler (1990) and Galinsky and Schopler (1994) also raised several potential harmful effects of SHGs. For those non-professionally-led groups, members may give misguided and misinformed information to one another. Regarding their peer leaders, if they are not professionally trained, they might not be able to effectively lead the group, for which they are not prepared. The condition may be even worse if they seek to provide therapy, such as the exploration of feelings, encouragement to examine interpersonal relationships within the group, and the like which could do harm than good to other members. Finally, SHGs the idea that may pressure newcomers to accept stigmatized identities and cult-like beliefs is another concern.

Though there are some potential problems in SHGs, which should be anticipated and dealt with when they arise, the general effectiveness of SHGs and the satisfaction reported by their members outweighs their potential problems. Some empirical studies on the effectiveness of SHGs will be reviewed in the next section.

7.9. Overseas Studies of SHGs

Powell (1985) did a good review of studies on both the professional support SHGs and autonomous SHGs, on or before the 1980s. The review showed that there were far more studies demonstrating the positive effects on SHGs than the negative ones. There were two representative studies showing negative findings. A study by Bankoff (1979) on widow groups, as an alternative to informal social support, showed that the acutely bereaved did not benefit. One possible explanation is they target the wrong problems or a lack of fit between the problem and the SHG. As suggested by Powell (1985), an individual suffering from acute problems could hardly benefit from an SHG whose primary purpose is for long-term mutual support and people may benefit only after the acute condition. The study on TOPS (Take Off Pounds Sensibly) by Garb and Stunkard (1974) found that when short-term members were followed up, many of those who lost small amounts of weight regained weight after leaving the organization, thus lowering the success rate substantially. As proposed by Powell (1985), one of the reasons of the negative findings of Stunkard's study was the defects of cross-sectional studies. Stunkard's early designs over-sampled long-term members and under-sampled short-term members, resulting in an over-estimation of the benefits of SHGs. Therefore, it is recommended to have longitudinal designs for evaluating the effectiveness of the SHG.

However, Powell (1985) has raised several difficulties relating to the evaluation of the effectiveness of SHGs. Firstly, it is difficult to study SHGs in an experimental design, which has experimental and control groups with randomized samplings, since it is impossible to define an appropriate sampling frame. Secondly, even with the time-series designs in which samples are being followed up for a long period of time without randomized control groups, there is the possibility that the outcome is affected by unmeasured variables outside the group. Finally, there is problem of construct validity to what extent the intervention is a sample of “true” self-help interventions, since the professionally supported SHG is different from the autonomous SHG with no professional involvement.

Rutchick (1990) also raised a number of problems in initiating research on a group's process in the health setting. Firstly, since an SHG has a small number of members, usually below 10, there is the problem of small sample size. When several groups are studied together in order to increase the sample size, goals, and structures of respective SHGs will increase sample variation. Secondly, research is confounded by the complexities of the group process and therapeutic change, which make it difficult to control variables. Complicating variables include individual characteristics of group members, such as pre-existing coping skills and personality traits, pre-group expectations and motivation, etc. Thirdly, the most complex and difficult to measure and control are group process variables. They are the characteristics that define and describe the interactions within a group such as cohesion, norms, group climate, role relationships, developmental stage etc. Finally, SHG’s research is hampered by the limited availability of practical and sound empirical measures that are not well developed.

Though there is paucity of group-practice research due to methodological issues, some recent studies on the effectiveness of SHGs are discussed as follows. A study by Grimsmo et al.,(1981) on a large-scale prospective study of over 10,000 people in a Norwegian SHG for weight reduction, found that there was significant and meaningful weight reduction which was retained over four years. Rothlis (1984) studied the effect of SHGs on feelings of hopelessness and helplessness by using a convenience sample of 28 patients with a primary diagnosis of reactive depression within six to twelve months of their hospitalization. They experienced a loss of an important person through death, divorce, or separation; a loss of job; a loss of status and prestige, such as church or other important organization membership; or a loss of part of the body such as a leg, or eyesight. The study utilized a pre-test, post-test control group design. Instruments used were the Beck Hopelessness Scale (HS) and Thornton’s Learned Helplessness Index (LHI). The findings supported that the exposure to SHG treatments would result in a significant decrease in feelings of hopelessness and helplessness in individuals with a diagnosis of reactive depression due to loss. Since all of the subjects were on various types and dosages of anti-depressants, it was difficult to determine the influence of these medications on the outcome. Due to the small size of the sample and population nature, generalizations can be made only to similar populations in psychiatric settings.

An empirical investigation of scoliosis peer support groups by Hinrichsen et al.,(1985) showed that members of SHGs experienced higher feelings of mastery and self-esteem. Lieberman and Videka-Sherman (1986) studied bereaved spouses who participated in SHGs, and compared to controls they showed a marked improvement in levels of depression, well-being, self-esteem, and life satisfaction. Toseland and Siporin (1986) in a review of 32 classical experimental design studies comparing individual and group treatment, found that in 75 percent of the studies, group treatment was as effective as individual treatment, and more effective in 25 percent. However, it had not addressed the question of who benefits under what conditions.

Trojan (1989) studied the benefits of SHGs as depicted by 232 members from 65 different disease-related groups by using closed-ended questionnaires. The focus of the study was on what the members reported about the changes and effects induced by their participation in SHGs. The effects of participation were grouped into the following categories. 1) Impact on disease-related stress (positive health effects, general enlargement of competence, general social activation). 2) Impact on the relationship with family and friends (relationship with partner, changes in personal network). 3) Impact on patient behavior and professional services (general enlargement of competence and social activation in relation to the professional care system, utilization of professional services). Most of the members reported considerable positive changes in these dimensions. However, which disease-related group reported more benefit outcome was not depicted in that study.

Another study by Wetzel (1991) investigated the strengths and limitations of SHGs for people and families with bipolar and unipolar illness. He used a convenience sample of 221 patients and relatives during a period of 2 years of participant observation. The findings showed that discussion of urgent illness-related problems was the most frequent, economical, and successful activity. Speigel (1993) organized SHGs as an intervention program for women with cancer and found that participants in a weekly discussion group lived longer on average than a control group.

Humphreys and Noke (1997) conducted a recent study on the influence of post-treatment mutual-help group participation on the friendship networks of substance-abuse patients. A convenience sample of a 1-year longitudinal study examining such effects in a sample of 237 male substance-abuse inpatients showed that 57.7% of whom became significantly involved in 12-step activities (e.g. reading program literature, attending meetings) after treatment. A priori model of the interplay of the 12-step involvement and friendship networks was tested using structural equation modeling, and found to have an excellent fit to the data. The twelve-step group involvement after treatment predicted better general friendship characteristics (e.g. number of close friends) and substance abuse-specific friendship characteristics (e.g. proportion of friends who abstain from drugs and alcohol) at follow-up.

With 388 SHG representatives randomly selected from over 2,000 groups in Kansas, Wituk et al.,(2000) successfully conducted telephone interviews on 253 SHG representatives to examine professional involvement, the members, and group characteristics. It was found that many SHGs have shared leadership and receive assistance from professionals and guidance from national and local organizations.

A case demonstration by Kohoe (2007) showed that spirituality groups specializing in serious mental illness help explore the spiritual beliefs and values of clients, which is a more holistic approach to the treatment of individuals with serious mental illness. It is suggested that people with serious mental illness search for the meaning of their experiences and look for hope, and many find both meaning and hope in their spiritual or religious beliefs and practices.

Dadich (2007) conducted interviews with 53 young people suffering diagnosable mental illness or substance abuse issues to explore their experiences with SHGs. They collectively represented 17 distinct SHGs and involved from their respective groups for 2.31 years with average attendance to 7.4 meetings per month. The qualitative results suggest that most of the young people found opportunities for spiritual growth through the SHGs, which they have involved with.

A comparison study was conducted by Peterson et al.,(2009) with 259 adults diagnosed as having a binge eating disorder. Samples were randomly assigned to 20 weeks of therapist-led, therapist-assisted, or self-help, or a waiting list group. Although results show that the therapist-led group did better, the lack of group differences at follow-up suggests that the self-help group approach may be a viable alternative treatment.

Overall, empirical research in health related group is limited, as most studies of SHGs have shown to be remarkably effective in promoting the recovery and rehabilitation of individuals who share common problems.

However, there were some methodological limitations in these studies. Firstly, some studies were with small sample sizes. Secondly, multiple methods have been used for these studies.

7.10. Local Studies of SHGs

Not until the end of the twentieth century were there some studies on SHGs in Hong Kong. Most studies were mainly focused on patients suffering from chronic physical illness. Only a few were done on mental patients.

In the mental healthcare settings, Ma's (1986) study was the first attempt to do research on the mutual-aid group as a practice model in working with the family members of psychotic patients. It was a qualitative evaluation focusing on both SHG's process and outcome. One of the relatives' groups with 3 months running led by the mutual aid group leaders was content-analyzed. Pre-group and post-group interviews with open-ended questions were conducted on the group process and the participants' change in the cognitive, affective, and behavioral domains. Results showed that mutual sharing, mutual support, and information giving were three significant elements characterizing the group process. However, no evidence was found to support that the program brought tremendous change to the participants' cognitive, affective, and behavioral domains. Though it was a good start in studying SHGs, there were several limitations in this research. Firstly, there were only 13 participants successfully interviewed, the number was too small for generalization. Secondly, there was no control group, so it was difficult to draw a conclusion without comparison to those who have not joined any SHG. Thirdly, no reliability checks were conducted on the content analysis. Finally, no long-term follow-up study was carried out afterwards to draw any conclusive remark on the exact effect of the change of the participants.

Ma (1992) also did a comprehensive review of mutual-aid groups for the mentally ill and their family members. It was found that there were only 3 SHGs for the mentally ill and no formal evaluation had been conducted. In the time of the present study, all these SHGs had stopped functioning. Difficulties identified to keep the continuity of the service include: lack of lay leaders; rapid turn-over of the project social worker; limited resources for future development; inadequate government support and skeptical responses from mental health professionals. However, it was predicted SHGs would be an effective, economical, and legitimate alternative for the community care of the mentally ill and their family members. The review also suggested that mental health professionals should be prepared to take up the challenge to bring SHGs to their members for greater benefits. Furthermore, Ma recommended to launch a summative evaluation research to study the effectiveness of these SHGs, unfortunately, none was conducted afterwards. Finally, she raised the issue of the need for policy makers and mental health professionals to change their philosophical orientation from consumerism to empowerment, and from being paternalistic to being democratic, which is essential for the long-term development of SHGs in Hong Kong.

Chan et al.,(1992) had carried out a local study on the impact of SHGs on chronically ill patients. Chan's study focused on identifying existing SHGs for individuals with chronic illness in Hong Kong, and aimed to make recommendations to government on rehabilitation, as well as on health and welfare policies. They identified 16 SHGs for people with chronic physical illness in Hong Kong through a snow-ball method. Then, questionnaire surveys plus long interviews were used to obtain information from 72 of the core group members who were patients or family members of these self-help organizations. The findings included information on the needs of individuals with chronic illness and the existing conditions of the SHGs among these patients and their families. A series of recommendations were also proposed to the Health and Welfare Branch. The study had not addressed the sampling method and thc validity of the instrument. Furthermore, those respondents' educational level was above average. It was possible that the more educated person was ready to participate in self-help activities and expressed their needs. Clearly, there were a large number of individuals with chronic illness not included in that study. Yet, it is the result of this research project that the Government has paid more attention in allocating resources to furthering the development of SHGs for chronically ill patients. It has also aroused concern among healthcare professionals in the hospitals to set up various SHGs.

Another study conducted by Wong (1993) explored the current situation of the self-help movement in Hong Kong and identified the factors affecting professional involvement, as well as differences in the working conditions between self-help organizations and service organizations. She used semi-structured interviews for a purposeful sampling of 21 respondents who were either social-work professionals or members drawn from two self-help organizations, and two service organizations for parents of the mentally-handicapped people or for physically-handicapped people. The findings concluded that the self-help movement demonstrated social significance in the society as it engaged in different activities to solve various problems in the social service provision, which resulted from poor community care. However, the findings could not be generalized due to the small sample size.

Mok (1998), a nursing professor, developed a model of empowerment for cancer patients and examined the role of SHGs in the empowering process. She combined in-depth interviews, participant-observation, and measurement development to capture the empowering aspects of the illness in a form that lent itself to quantitative analysis. Her study was comprehensive by combining qualitative and quantitative methods, in that the concepts could be meaningfully and carefully examined, and a systematic comparison was possible. Yet, the constructed model of empowerment only suited the cancer patients while other disease groups were not addressed.

Another study was conducted by Mok (2001) on the effectiveness of an SHG from the members' own perception. The study adopted a cross-sectional survey design, supplemented by qualitative in-depth interviews and participant observation. One hundred SHGs were randomly selected from 211 SHGs identified from all social welfare agencies and hospitals in Hong Kong. 719 valid self-administered questionnaires were completed by their members. In addition, in-depth interviews and participant observation were carried out with 10 groups which were divided into four major types: groups for physical illness, mental illness, physically and mentally disabled and marginal group, such as single parents and families on welfare etc. The findings indicated participation in SHGs could lead to very positive psychological changes for individuals and also generate tremendous psychosocial, and even material, benefit for members.

Chien et al.,(2005) conducted a randomized controlled trial to examine the effectiveness of a 12-session mutual support group for Chinese families caring for a relative with schizophrenia compared with a psycho-educational group and routine family support services in Hong Kong. Families were randomly assigned to receive mutual support (n=32), psycho-education (n=33) or standard care only (n=31). Pre and post tests on families' functioning, mental health service utilization, patients' level of functioning, and duration of re-hospitalization were measured. Results showed that family caregivers and patients in the mutual support group had significant improvements in the outcome measures than other groups. The findings support the effectiveness of mutual support groups as a means to improve both family and patient functioning. When an 18-month follow-up study was conducted (Chien et al., 2006), results showed that mutual support consistently produced greater improvement in patient and family functioning, and caregiver burden over the intervention and follow-up periods, compared with the other two conditions.

The findings further support the effectiveness of mutual support in helping families of Chinese people with schizophrenia.

All in all, a literature review of the recent two decades of local studies of SHGs in Hong Kong shows that few studies are conducted on mental patients. Despite the fact that a successful SHG must be ongoing and long-term, as most problems faced by former psychiatric patients are chronic in nature and require ongoing support or care (Lamb, 1986), no long-term SHGs for psychotic patients was developed in the past. Until the establishment of a recent one run by Christian Oi Hip Fellowship, which is the target organization for this book, there is only one self-help organization with a long-term SHG for mental patients. Furthermore, except some SHGs with religious elements for drug rehabilitation locally, only few programs with integrated spiritual dimension are for psychiatric patients, and no comprehensive review has been carried out on the effectiveness of these programs.

7.11. Existing Policy of Self-Help in Hong Kong

There are policy statements stressing the importance of social support networks and self-help among citizen groups; and to instill a patient-oriented culture or service, with greater community participation so that providers are more in touch with the users' need (Hong Kong Government, 1991; Hong Kong Government, 1993). In the Chapter on "Philosophy and General Provision of Social Welfare" of the 1991 White Paper, the role of social networks is highlighted. The contributions of social networks in the service provision are much emphasized. The following claims were stated in the White Paper (Hong Kong Government, 1991).

> "It has been stated that social welfare services should be made available to all who need them. However, such an objective cannot be achieved without the support of an input from the community through the establishment of networks of informal care and support provided by families, friends and neighbors. Such networks, together with the more formal services, aim at helping people to achieve maximum independence and maintain control over their own lives.
>
> Social networks are part of Chinese culture and tradition and have always existed in Hong Kong. They are most clearly demonstrated in the role of the family as the primary provider of care and welfare and by the contributions of clansmen associations, neighborhood organizations and

volunteers. Recent years have seen the more structured and conscious promotion of the concept of social workers and community organizers in the setting up of support groups and self-help groups.

Providing care and support through social networks will be developed and nurtured and it will be necessary to map out the principal objectives and providing supporting services and facilities for the care givers involved. The development of this concept of service delivery does not imply any entrenchment of responsibilities on the part of Government in the provision of services. Rather, it is the development of an approach within the existing and future infrastructure which will allow more choice for service recipients and encourage greater self-reliance." (p. 18)

Despite the claims on the importance of social networks in the Social Welfare White Paper, neither are concrete programs proposed on strengthening existing networks, nor recommendations made to set up new networks for social support. Social support for the psychiatric patient is particularly crucial as studies showed that people with strong social support enjoy better mental health and their rate of utilizing mental health services is significantly reduced (Becker et al., 1997; Hamilton et al., 1989; Scherbourne, 1988).

According to the Rehabilitation Green Paper 1992, self-help was recognized as an important component of rehabilitation for individuals with disabilities or chronic illness. It was mentioned that SHGs should be encouraged and promoted, as group members could give psychological support and comfort to each other by sharing their own experiences (Hong Kong Government, 1992). On the other hand, Government support for SHGs has not been specified in those papers. In the Hong Kong Rehabilitation Program Plan (Hong Kong Government 1999), the contributions of self-help organizations are once again recognized and the Government strongly supports the further development of the self-help organizations. But, the Social Welfare Department will only provide the necessary support and assistance to self-help organizations in their application for premises, as appropriate.

"Apart from providing meaningful social, educational and leisure activities, self-help organizations promote a spirit of mutual help among people with disabilities as well as their parents/careers. These organizations also represent people with disabilities to express their views on rehabilitation services, to service providers and government departments concerned. Through seminars, campaigns and the mass media, self-help organizations foster a positive image of and promote the rights of people with disabilities" (p. 174).

Furthermore, it is clearly stated that the Government will not provide any financial support in any staffing expenses and operational costs.

> "Self-help organizations have been requesting the Government to provide financial assistance to support their staffing expenses and operational costs. However, under existing subvention policy, the Government will only sub vent the operational costs associated with provision of certain direct welfare services" (p. 174).

Social networks are part of the Chinese culture and tradition, and have always existed in Hong Kong. One of the examples, are those neighborhood organizations. However, the former psychiatric patients are still strongly stigmatized and limited support and attention has been raised by the community.

7.12. Self-Help Organizations in Hong Kong

There is a major expansion in the scientific aspects on the self-help phenomenon globally, and apparently there is a significant rise in the occurrence of self-help throughout the world (Gidron & Chesler, 1994). However, the development in Hong Kong is rather slow especially in the mental health setting. As suggested by Wong and Chan (1994), there is a strong sense of professional paternalism in which doctors dominate the treatment process and patients are submissive to the professional authority. Patient involvement is minimal since patient - doctor interaction and communication is inadequate. The notion of self-responsibility and mutual support among patients is largely undermined in the present healthcare system.

Chronically-ill individuals and their families require assistance and support in coping with difficulties arising from their illness. In mid-1993, the Hong Kong Society for Rehabilitation and other non-governmental organizations drew up a proposal for implementing a pilot scheme called, "Community Rehabilitation Network (CRN)". With the support from the Government, the project received a grant from the Royal Hong Kong Jockey Club for the setting up of a clearing house and two CRN centers for a trial period of 18 months. These facilities came into operation in early 1994 (Hong

Kong Government, 1995). CRN aims to enhance the quality of life for people with visceral disability and their families by giving them support, mutual-help groups, social networking, and educational activities. It provides a meeting place for them to share and learn experiences and skills in managing their daily life. From April 1997, one clearing house and three CRN centers have been operating with subvention (Hong Kong Government, 1998). Owing to manpower and resource limitations, CRN has to begin the service with selected patient groups, and former psychiatric patients are not included. It was thought that former psychiatric patients are well taken care of by those non-government organizations working for the mentally ill, such as Baptist Oi Kwan Social Service and the Richmond Fellowship, Hong Kong. But in fact, no long-term SHGs for the mentally ill were really developed at that time.

With the self-help movement, and encouragement and help from the health professionals, when patients and family members start to communicate with one another, the SHGs can be formed quite easily. However, without continuous administrative support, the groups may remain at an informal level for a long time or even indefinitely. Chan et al.,(1996) identified 62 SHGs among patients in Hong Kong. Yet, there is no SHG for the former psychiatric patients on the list.

The first SHG for the mentally ill people was the "Friends of Lok Kwan Psychiatric Half-way House" of "Baptist Oi Kwan Social Service", which was started by the aftercare workers and the volunteers of Baptist Oi Kwan Social Service in 1986 (Yiu & Ng, 1989). Other groups are provided by the Hong Yee and Fok Yee Club of the Hong Kong Family Welfare Society started in 1987 for the graduates of the cognitive behavioral groups run by the same agents that suffered from minor mental health problems, such as adjustment difficulty or mild depression. Following this, some of the social workers and aftercare workers of the half-way houses also started to organize SHGs for their residents (Ma, 1992). Now, only the groups of Hong Kong Family Welfare Society continue to operate, those groups in the half-way houses became loosely organized with the departure of the aftercare worker.

The Hang Hong Mutual Aid Group was established in May 1996 by a group of former psychiatric patients. The Happy Sharing Group and the Kai Hong Club for former psychiatric patients was established in Nov, 1997 and Oct, 1999, respectively, with the help of community psychiatric nurses.

These groups are usually run by some core members who are responsible for the planning and the implementation of the activities for the less active members, while the professionals would act as consultants and provide advice whenever necessary. Members of these groups meet regularly. These groups are open groups and welcome new members at any time. The activities of these groups are mainly educational and recreational in nature, in the form of educational talks, small group discussions, parties, outings, camping, home visits, and publication of newsletters. No counseling service is provided for their members but rather by participating in the above-mentioned activities, they could receive more information and emotional support from one another.

It is a good sign having more SHGs developed within the former psychiatric patient field. However, they are confronting a lot of problems. Firstly, there is a lack of peer leaders. Some active members are quite energetic in the initial stage of forming the SHG, but after a period of time, they may find that it is too stressful to be leaders all the time and become burnout. They may not have prepared successors when they change their role to become less active and that can lead to the failure of maintaining the group for a long time. Secondly, Mok (2001) in his study of the effectiveness of SHGs found that SHG involvement could result in both positive and negative experiences. The negative impact included pressure felt to conform to group demands, feeling uncomfortable and useless in the group. Therefore, how the leader leads the group is one of the key factors affecting .success. The study by Schopler and Galinsky (1981) suggests that leadership is one of the most important factors related to negative interactions. In addition to leadership, Smokoski et al.,(2001) pointed out that members' attribution and actions, such as reluctance to participate and a poor fit to the group were also important factors associated with negative group experiences. Finally, since there is no support from the government in terms of resources in encouraging the intervention of SHGs in psychiatric rehabilitation, input from the professional staff is quite limited with the stringent resources in all non-government organizations. Not surprisingly, without strong peer leadership and enough professional involvement, the nature of the group content is quite confined to social activities without any well-structured program.

On the contrary, though lack of peer leaders is also a problem facing the Fellowship, there are professional staff members that are all Christian volunteers in the groups. Their religious beliefs strengthen their commitment in the group, which maintains a partnership model and keeps the group going in the long run. Professional staff members, also help develop a norm within the consensus of the group. Besides these, a structured program including skill learning and a peer leader supported retreat is designed to train group members to become peer leaders. An annual retreat is organized for all the professional volunteers to boost morale and training. With reinforcement to both peer leaders and professional volunteers, the first SHG in the Fellowship has been running for more than 20 years. The Fellowship will be introduced in details in the next section.

7.13. THE FOCUS ORGANIZATION OF THIS BOOK: THE CHRISTIAN OI HIP FELLOWSHIP

The Christian Oi Hip Fellowship, described below as the Fellowship, is a self-help organization, initiated by a Christian former psychiatric patient and formed with the help from a hospital chaplain and some Christian mental-health professionals including psychiatrists, nurses, social workers, and occupational therapists. The founders of the Fellowship were Mr. Mak Fun Yu (ex-patient), Reverend Chan Yi Wah (hospital chaplain) and Mr. Andrew Leung LUK (psychiatric nurse). When adopting the classification by Levine and Perkins (1987), the Fellowship was the first type of SHG that is made up of former psychiatric patients with stigmatizing conditions. The Fellowship has reached the last stage of growth of an SHG as classified by Katz (1970), and has established a formal organization with full-time professional staff. The Fellowship was one of the pioneers in organizing SHGs for former psychiatric patients. It is a beneficiary of the "Community Chest", a charitable organization from which the Fellowship receives its fund for part of the expenditure. The rest of the funding relies mainly on the donations of professionals, churches, volunteers, and members.

Organization History (Oi Hip Fellowship, 2000)

In early 1989, a Christian former psychiatric patient deeply felt the need for social support when he had to face many challenges in the community during rehabilitation, so he started a network with those of the same background. With the help from some Christian mental-health professionals and a hospital chaplain, the first SHG for male former psychiatric patients was started with regular meetings. Starting from the middle of 1989, the group held monthly meetings. In 1990, the gatherings increased to twice a month. On June 1990, it was named as Christian Oi Hip Fellowship. In August of the same year, a female group was formed. Since then, all other groups formed are of mixed sex so that members can learn how to interact with the opposite sex as they would do in society.

In early 1991, it was registered as a non-profit organization. Starting from 1994, the Fellowship held courses on mental health to educate the public on mental illness and the ways to cope with it. In early 1995, a volunteer committee consisting of 4 working groups: witness group, newsletter group, visiting group, and activity group was established. The aim of this committee was to provide the group members with opportunities to participate in social service and become helpers in the future.

In February 1996, a resource center was set up to provide information services, books and magazine lending service, and an audio-visual lending service to the members and the public. In August 1996, the Annual General Meeting passed the motion of establishing a Pastoral Care Committee to foster the growth of the member's spiritual life and faith. In May1998, through the grant from the CWM/Nethersole Fund, the organization bought a permanent site as the premises for the organization.

Organizational objectives and service areas

The organization is a non-profit Christian organization that emphasizes on mutual support. The objectives are as follows:

1. To provide "holistic care" for former psychiatric patients. Holistic care is defined as a philosophy and practice of compassionate care, which respects the value and dignity of man and upholds the physical, psychological, social, and spiritual well-being of the total person.
2. To establish an effective support system and reduce the chance of relapse.
3. To help churches in caring for former psychiatric patients. Many former psychiatric patients would seek spiritual assistance from local churches, which sometimes find it difficult to accommodate them into the religious group owing to their problems in rehabilitation. Therefore, churches are one of the target organizations for the Fellowship's service in terms of providing consultation, training and referrals.
4. To help the ex-patients to re-integrate into the society and churches.
5. To promote mental health education.

With the support of the "Community Chest", a charity foundation, the organization has not only been working actively for the welfare of the members, but also promoting services to the community as a whole. The service areas can be broadly classified into five main areas as follows:

1. **Personal Care**
   To emphasize on individual needs, help clients to grow and change, provide home visits, and counseling.

2. **Group Work**
   To emphasize on mutual support in belief and daily living and encourage them to be independent and to help each other.

3. **Consultation and training**
   To assist churches in caring for ex-patients, provide consultation services and promote mental health education to the general public.

4. **Communal activities**
   To provide classes on other interests and outdoor activities so as to improve members' social skills and the quality of life.

5. **Former psychiatric patients' resource center**
   To promote mental health and psychiatric public education, as well as provide members with more knowledge and resources to cope with their problems.

Organization Structure

The organization structure is presented in the organization chart in Appendix 1. All the posts stated are voluntary in nature except the staff team that consists of one assistant social-welfare officer, two pastors, one social-work assistant, and one clerical staff. There are two types of membership in the Fellowship. The first one is client membership for former psychiatric patients who are willing to join in the SHG for personal growth. They need not to have any religious beliefs but are open to participate in a Christian spiritual practice i.e. prayer. The second one is professional membership for Christian mental-health professionals who are willing to serve the special target group of former psychiatric patients. They are all volunteers including psychiatrists, psychiatric nurses, psychiatric social workers, occupational therapists, and hospital chaplains who act mostly as group counselors. Other volunteers who are not mental health professionals are required to attend training programs provided by the Fellowship prior to their service to the clients. The training programs include courses on stress management, common psychiatric disorders, psychiatric rehabilitation, and clinical placement. In the year 2000, there were 12 SHGs in this Fellowship which became a leading self-help organization for former psychiatric patients in Hong Kong.

Philosophy

Since it is a Christian organization, the Fellowship holds the belief that it is established and maintained with the governance of God. So that everyone in the Fellowship, including the professionals and group members, can help one another, and have personal growth in the love of God. The name "Oi Hip" in Chinese means, "In the love of God we help each other." The mission of the Fellowship is 'in the love of God, we help ourselves and one another to live an abundant life.' An abundant life in the Biblical context is a holistic approach with physical, psychological, social, and spiritual fullness. Therefore, it is a partnership model in partnership with God, and with one another to live to one's fullness.

Based on the Biblical background, the Fellowship holds five core values that it believes to be valuable to both the professional and client members for personal growth. The core values are as follows:

1. We are all valuable individuals created by God
   (Genesis: 1:27; Psalm 8: 4-5; John 3:16)
   Since we are valued in the eye of God, we believe that we have good self-worth, self-image, and self-esteem that could not be taken away by anyone, not even by ourselves.

2. We are pardoned by God as we confess our sins and refrain from our wrong doing (Roman 5:1-2; II Cor 5: 17; John 1:9)
   Since we are forgiven by God, we should forgive anyone who has done wrong to us. We should live a guilt-free life.

3. We are known by God as Christ has once been human and understands us.
   (John 1:14; Hebrews 4: 15-16; I Cor 10:13)
   Since God empathizes with us, we are not alone when facing crisis in our lives.

4. We are surrounded by God's love as we are treasured by Him and nothing can separate us from Him (Matthew 10: 29-31; 11: 28-30; Roman 8:31-39) Since we are protected by God, we have joy and peace coming from within that is long lasting.

5. We can live an abundant life as God gives us strength (Philippians 4:13; Romans 8: 26; James 5:16) Since we are empowered by God, we have the strength to live a new life with hope through prayers and mutual support from one another.

Developing from the core values, 8 basic beliefs have been published in the Fellowship pamphlet.

1. God loves man.
2. Every individual is equal and valuable before God.
3. "Holistic care" embodies the care of one's physical, psycho, social, and spiritual aspects.
4. "Self-help" is the essential element for the rehabilitation and individual growth of the mentally ill.
5. The Fellowship can facilitate personal growth of the members (including staff workers, volunteers and the former psychiatric patients) through the love of God.
6. The Fellowship can help members experience the love of God through the application of Bible teachings in their lives, prayers, and mutual support.
7. Every member of the Fellowship is able to contribute towards the Fellowship.
8. The Fellowship can help the former psychiatric patients re-integrate into the community through God's love and mutual help.

Group Intervention

The time required to mature for each SHG in the Fellowship is expected to be within five years. It is a partnership model formed by both mental-health professionals and former psychiatric patients. During the formative stage, the professionals who are the group counselors would take a more active role and act as the leader and facilitator. After five years, when the SHG has matured, or is in a self-sustaining stage, the role of the group counselors would be changed, as group advisor with group members form their own planning committee for co-ordination and planning.

A group meeting is held once every fortnight. One meeting is for open-sharing and praying. Another meeting is used for sharing a special topic that concerns all members. In the first six months of an SHG, a manual for stress management is developed by the Fellowship is prepared for the group to use (Appendix 2). For the rest of the time, the group members themselves would initiate the sharing topic (Appendix 3). In some of the more mature groups, alongside regular meetings, there are some gatherings to initiate further bonding. Also, the Fellowship as a whole would organize regular outdoor activities, e.g. outings, camping, and retreats so that all group members can have more opportunities to understand one another and enlarge their social circle. The group intervention model is attached in Appendix 4.

Stages of group development

In the design of a new group in the Fellowship, the development of the group is roughly divided into four stages. The initial stage is the first 6 months of joining a group when a new member has to get familiar with the other members and the group norm. If it is a newly formed group, a standardized stress program developed by the Fellowship will be used. The second stage is development stage from 6 months to 2 years when one will develop trust of others if he or she can mix well in the group and becomes more involved in the group activities. The third stage is the mature stage from 2 to 5 years when members choose to stay behind and will usually be invited to be the committee members of their respective groups to learn to plan the group meetings and to care for the new comers. During this period, some groups can be independent and maintain their own activities without much involvement of the group counselors. The final stage is the self-sustaining stage when the group has been running for more than 5 years and develops its own programs or activities. Some key members of the group would maintain the norm of their respective groups and take an active role in caring for the new comers.

Chapter 8

Studies Related to the Effectiveness of the Holistic Care Program

A preliminary qualitative study conducted by Leung and Arthur (2004) on clients and facilitators of the program indicated members had positive experiences and some changes in their lives which contributed to the rehabilitation of their illness. Adopting a multi-method approach, LUK and Shek (2006a) first used a quasi-experimental design to evaluate the program and found that those who joined the program had more friends and more social satisfaction than the control subjects. Using a repertory grid based on the personal construct theory to measure self-identity changes after joining the program, LUK and Shek (2006b) found that participants perceived positive changes in physical, psychological, social, and spiritual dimensions after joining the program. In a qualitative approach, results showed that by attending the program, participants had positive feelings and gained many positive learning opportunities when interacting with peers. Interacting with group leaders was also very beneficial to them (LUK & Shek 2008). In this qualitative study, a total of 20 members from the program, which was about one sixth of all the regular group members, were recruited. In total there were 52 themes emerging from the data, 7, 23, and 22 from the structure, process, and outcome components, respectively. However, because of the focus of the research question (i.e., experiences in joining the program) and space limitation, only 13 themes on experience of the process component, which showed participants' experiences in SHGs and 9 themes on the personal changes of the outcome component which illustrated their perceived changes by attending the program were presented here. A summary of the themes in these two major categories is illustrated in Table 2. The details of the findings can also be seen in LUK (2004).

Table 2. A summary of themes in the major category of experiences in the group and perceived personal changes

Framework	Major categories	Sub-categories	Themes
Process	Experience	Uniqueness (the uniqueness of one's group)	Spiritual orientation Participation and caring group Group variation
		Experi_mem (experiences with group members)	Empathy Positive learning opportunities Positive feelings Dark side of the illness
		Experi_coun (experiences with group counselors)	Positive encounter Importance of group counselors Limitation of group counselors
		Impress_experi (the most impressive experiences in group)	Various support from members Support from group counselors Support from God
Outcome	Personal changes	Changephysi (changes physically)	Better physical health
		Changepsycho (changes psychologically)	Development of positive feeling Development of positive thinking Increase of self-esteem
		Changesocial (changes socially)	Improvement of interpersonal skills Increased number of friends
		Changespirit (changes spiritually)	Rediscovery of the meaning and purpose of life An improved relation with God Developing spiritual strength

Experiences in the Group

Regarding the experiences in the group, three themes emerged in the subcategories of the uniqueness of the group. The first theme that emerged was the 'spiritually-oriented group'. One participant noted that, "I have not attended church for a long time, in Oi Hip, I can pray, sing hymns and maintain attendance of some religious meetings." The second theme was the 'participating and caring group'. Words like involvement, cohesiveness, and solidarity all showed a strong participation of the group members. Besides, those words like warmth, understanding, mutual respect, and love signified a caring atmosphere between members of the group. One participant expressed, "our special feature is we are well united. Like xx and me, we understand each other very well. We are bonded together with the love of Christ." A second participant claimed that, "my group is quite relaxing. I have not joined other groups and not clear about them. I feel in this group, it is relaxing among the members and the counselors, seems to be quite peaceful." The third theme was 'groups with variation'. Since participants were from different groups, some contradicting characteristics of group members were identified. One participant noted that, "what is the difference? Few are weaker, mentally not well and have difficulties in thinking." Another participant responded, "I feel that Oi Hip members know how to avoid embarrassment in public settings. Because I have tried other groups, they would not ask embarrassing questions that is in public, and will say appropriate things in appropriate settings."

With reference to their experiences with other members, four themes emerged: The first theme that emerged was 'empathy'. They had a strong sense of being empathized with by their peers. One participant gave the following account, "we have a very good relationship among members. Because we are all ex-patients, we have similar feelings when we share." A second participant claimed that, "I feel very well. Because other people, that is those without this illness might not be so helpful. For example, even if the counselors, when I am not well, or, for some time, routinely taking sick leave, when talking to her, she tells me not to do it. When you take too much sick leave, at redundancy time, it will be your turn. I listen to her, but ultimately possibly get used to it, once not well, take sick leave. Sometimes, the counselors may not have so much time to talk to you, not for an hour, just a few words. I feel better to turn to group members." The second theme was 'positive learning opportunities'. During the experiences with their peers, they received feedback from friends who saw things from a different perspective, observed members who had positive changes and were encouraged, and made reference to those whose behavior was socially acceptable and encouraged in the group. All these could provide them with good learning opportunities. After that, they could practice what they learned in the group in real life situation. One participant noted that *X* group leader, "previously was rather passive and withdrawn, but he is willing to take up this job and every time he is better. One group member did not believe in the past but now has suddenly accepted Christ. He did not like attending the group before but now he would attend even if he is late. We are much encouraged by seeing this person changed." A second participant expressed that, "Once, our counselor asked us to write something about one another for encouragement. One sister wrote, 'You are very gentle and quiet. Do concentrate on finding a job.' I thought I was not that quiet. My mother always said that I was very rude but she said I was very gentle and quiet. I thought I was like a little of what she said." The third theme was 'positive feelings'. Having the same background together with a relaxed and protective environment in the group setting, they felt free to disclose their views and feelings. Nearly all of them felt good and had a positive feeling towards their members. One participant depicted, "I feel quite close to the group members and our relationship is better than my relationship with other people. It is probably because we know we are all ex-mentally ill, I don't need to hide so many things and can easily be more frankly in our interaction." A second participant claimed, "We are friends and can support each other. We are in the same boat and can care for each other." The fourth theme was the 'dark side of the illness'. Some negative aspects such as, sensitivity to other people and passivity in social interaction, which were commonly seen in chronic mental patients were expressed by some participants. One participant noted that members have lower self-image and lack of self-confidence. Sometimes, when they are asked to try leading a meeting, they will probably say they are incapable. A second participant responded, "I remember that I once had some argument with a sister." In fact, that sister was having a relapse.

In their experiences with group counselors, three themes emerged. The first theme that emerged was the 'positive encounters' with the group counselors who sincerely developed friendships with them. With the therapeutic relationship, they felt they were being cared for, respected, and supported. They also showed appreciation for what they have done for them. One participant depicted that, "the counselors are quite nice. They really care about you and you can tell them your concerns. They also tell me what is right and what is wrong." Another expressed, "a few of us walk to the railway station, which is quite far away, together. We talk while walking and on the train. There are no barriers in between, that is, we are like friends." The second theme was the 'importance of group counselors' in the mutual support group. Beyond providing guidance and acting as a problem solver, the roles of a mediator were well demonstrated. As professionals in the mutual support group, they were in a better position to solve disagreements or conflicts between members with their knowledge and neutrality in the group. One participant noted, "They are willing to respond to any of my questions. About topical discussion, that's very good, because I benefit a lot through discussion with them on how to present the topic. When it comes to actual problems in my life, it is very good to have support from the counselors." A second participant claimed, "I was wronged about something. Then, I was unhappy and got into a quarrel in one meeting. The counselor then mediated. I used to think counselors are not very important because they seemed to be passive in their caring. After this incidence, I feel the counselors are active and both counselors are good, stop our quarrel promptly, separate us, so that everyone can cool down. They then attempt to analyze the problem. Afterwards, I realized that sister was admitted to hospital and then she might be not well at that time." The third theme was the perceived 'limitations of the group counselors'. They understood that sometimes the group counselors could not spend much time with them individually. One participant responded "when you have any problem and worry, it is helpful to talk to them. However, I think there's lack of time, cannot follow up that much.... That is they are rather busy, can't bother them once, and then the next time." A second participant claimed that, "sometimes, I feel as if a son is asking the mother, she sounds relatively at the top and I myself at the bottom, but it is still acceptable."

With regard to their most impressive experiences, the main theme that emerged was the 'various supports from peers' in terms of encounters with positive feelings, which were consistent with their general experiences with their peers who offered empathy and positive learning opportunities. One participant noted that they remembered, "January this year, I had just been discharged from hospital and was not very happy then because of the feeling why I was repeatedly going in and out of hospital. The group meeting that day happened to be sharing. I expressed my feelings and many counselors and members comforted me. I felt deeply impressed by that incident." A second participant claimed, "One member called xxx, who has been attending the group for about 2 years, is good at caring. He sends birthday cards to other members on their birthdays. When I am feeling down, he sends me cards with scriptural verses to encourage me. It gave me an unforgettable impression." The second theme was the 'support from group counselors' who showed their integrity and earned their respect. Furthermore, they could really provide practical guidance and help to them. One participant expressed that, "I was leading a spiritual sharing. I could not remember what I said at the time, but the young counselor watched me seemingly as if she was watching her children getting a prize in a prize presentation ceremony and her eye contact was so encouraging. It made me feel I was not abandoned." A second participant responded, "I remembered that once I was very down, I talked to the counselor. He comforted me and I talked to him a few more times after that. But I realized that I needed to tackle the problems by myself afterwards. I changed from dependence at an early stage to taking some action after talking and listening to the opinion given. I feel it really helps me practically, including whether you believe or not, listen first." The third theme was the 'support from God'. God's love was sensed via the interaction of members in the group. One participant depicted that, "once or twice when I led songs, I felt a relatively stronger spiritual atmosphere. The message of the songs would touch the hearts of the members. Although we are a deprived group, God loves us and cares about us, and leads us in our lives and work. One other time, we had a gathering at Mr Xx's home. We had dinner together and sharing, were much able to experience the taste of the love of Jesus and the love for one another."

PERCEIVED PERSONAL CHANGES

Where physical changes after participation in the groups are concerned, only one theme emerged, 'better physical health', since not many specific changes were identified by participants. One participant expressed, "I feel the appetite become better. Possibly the problem in the mind is solved."

With respect to psychological changes after participation in the groups, three themes emerged: The first theme that emerged was the 'development of positive feelings'. After joining the group, the new members knew that they were not alone and were even better than others. Besides, they had time for ventilation and even received support from one another. All these made them feel happier. One participant noted, "I have learned to be cheerful. I know some members are very supportive. Comparatively, many of their situations are no better than me but they are stronger. I have learned from them." A second participant claimed, "I have got to know some friends. I then realize that I am not alone and there are a group of people like me. This makes me feel better psychologically." The second theme was the 'development of positive thinking'. When mixing well in the group, they received support and were encouraged. They developed more positive thinking towards their illnesses and lives. One participant responded, "I am more positive and not as pessimistic as before." A second participant expressed, "I am more open to a lot of things. As I get to know more members through activities of Oi Hip with mutual support and I become more positive and optimistic in facing this illness." The final theme was the 'increase of self-esteem'. This helps in the respect that being a member of a group, having a better health condition than some members, being respected, appreciated, recognized by others, knowing more friends, and having some contribution in the group by either being a committee member or giving support to others, would more-or-less increase their sense of self-worth and enhanced their self-esteem. One participant depicted that, "I am less feeling of inferiority. Together, we are all the same. I am not the worst. Some are even in a worse situation." A second participant described, "I feel the group has re-established my ability to socialize. The group members accept me and show appreciation. That means I am loved, respected, appreciated and affirmed. That's why this is important to me. I feel this is the most important thing for joining Oi Hip, the most precious thing that I gain most."

When considering changes socially after participation in the group, two themes emerged. The first theme that emerged was the 'improvement of interpersonal skills'. They learned the positive skills like taking active role to interact with others, openness, expressive, being kind, caring, trusting others, avoid being too critical, and to control one's talkativeness. One participant claimed that, "I was very passive previously and only took action when pushed. Now I take initiative to show concern towards others. A second participant responded that I have learned here to be less critical about others. If I am kind to others, other will be kind to you too." The second theme was the 'increased number of friends'. After joining the group, they became familiar with one another. Based on a common background, members could develop friendships more easily and some could even develop a close relationship with a number of group members. One participant expressed, "Perhaps, I did not know them before but now became friends. He would chat to you when he had time. You wished the day of meeting would come sooner, Thursday would come sooner, and you were eager to attend the group."

With regard to changes spiritually, three themes emerged. The first theme that emerged was the 'rediscovery of meaning and purpose of life'. Before joining the group, they were very much affected by their illnesses that hindered their personal development. After accepting their limitations, they faced their lives more positively and some could find a role in the group as a healthy model. One participant noted that, "The meaning of life! I used to have strong emphasis on money but now it is not so important. I feel money is not the most important. Love, fruit of the spirit or family relationship are more important." A second participant claimed, "I was not sure about my goal of life before joining Oi Hip. Now, it seems I have discovered an important goal. I was sick and have now recovered. With the grace of God, I can live a normal life and work. I can live a life which is physically and mentally well, active, positive, hopeful, and joyful. I can tell other group members that they can also live such a life with God's grace." The second theme was 'an improved relationship with God'. With better communication with their God through reading bible, frequent prayer, there was growth in one's faith and the relationship with God has improved. One participant responded, "I have talked more to Him and would tell Him many other things. A second participant expressed that, "My relationship with God has improved, I become more dependent on Him and my faith has also increased." The last theme was 'developing spiritual strength'. With the spiritual awareness and the change of perception of God, who was loving and caring and had not deserted them in times of illness, they could find strength to live a better life and maintained a good bonding with their God. One participant depicted that, "I used to feel that God was very harsh. Now I feel He is not that harsh and is not mindful about my shortcomings, weaknesses, and sins." A second participant said, "My relationship with God has improved immensely. I try to pray, read the Bible or spiritual books daily. I feel full of energy and preach the gospel to other people because I am in debt to God. God has given me so much and I feel I should give Him something in return by preaching the gospel, introducing people to Oi Hip or sharing with others."

LUK (2011) conducted a follow up study to investigate the long-term effects of the holistic care program. Perception of help from the program and factors relating to the outcomes of the program were also studied. The study was intended to investigate the long-term effects of this holistic care program for individuals with serious mental illness after the last study conducted 5 years ago (LUK & Shek 2006a). Basically, the questions posed in that study were: Is the program still effective after 5 years' time? What are the subjective perceptions of the benefits gained from the program by the participants? What are the factors relating to the outcome measures? A quantitative approach using a set of self-administered questionnaires was adopted. The data was compared to a quasi-experimental study conducted in 2003 by LUK and Shek, involving an experimental group and a control group (LUK & Shek 2006a). Results showed that all the outcome measures of participants were similar to that of the experimental group found in last study. When compared with the control group, it was found that the participants had more hope than the control subjects. Help perceived from the program included support, encouragement, enhancement of self-confidence, spiritual assistance, and reflection of values. Having a job is found to be a key factor in relating to the outcomes of the program participants. The study concluded that the program is effective in providing some positive changes to its participants. Help is perceived by most participants and the program is also useful to provide mutual support to participants in maintaining a job in the community, which is a paramount factor for rehabilitation. All these studies relating to the effectiveness of the holistic program held by the Fellowship demonstrated that a partnership model in SHGs seems to be successful in providing support for the rehabilitation of people with serious mental illness. The spiritual element should be incorporated into psychiatric rehabilitation program to instill hope and meaningfulness of life. Nurses should be better educated in providing holistic care to individual clients and to a group.

Chapter 9

CONCLUSION

THEORETICAL AND PRACTICAL IMPLICATIONS OF THE HOLISTIC CARE PROGRAM

There were several theoretical implications of the evidences shown by the Fellowship. Firstly, regarding the SHG, the program provided more theoretical grounds for the small group theory. The themes developed in the qualitative case studies about the experiences of members such as "empathy", "positive learning opportunities", and "positive feelings" supported the previous studies of therapeutic forces available in small groups (Rutchick, 1990; Yalom, 1970). The findings of both studies by LUK and Shek (2006a; 2008) supported the previous findings that there was the need of the long-term nature of SHGs in providing continuous intervention to the chronically-ill patients (Gartner & Riessman, 1982; Lamb, 1986). They also supported the consistent findings of the essential components of participation and empowerment that could effect change in the SHG in the literature on small group studies (Hardiman & Segal, 2003; Riessman & Gartner, 1987; Segal, Silverman, & Temkin, 1993).

Secondly, this holistic care program supports the strengths of the mixed research method. The study by LUK and Shek (2006a) using the non-equivalent control group yielded objective data. However, the scope of the findings was quite narrow in terms of testing the hypotheses. On the other hand, the findings in LUK and Shek (2008)'s qualitative approach using the in-depth interviews yielded subjective data. Though the data were from the subjective experiences of the informants, they provided a broader view and fruitful information about the SHG. The findings in LUK and Shek (2006b) (Repertory Grid Method) provided additional quantitative and qualitative data to support the findings. By triangulation of all the quantitative and qualitative data, a comprehensive view on the changes of the participants in the program could be obtained. Finally, all studies about the Fellowship added to the database on SHGs and holistic care in mental health settings, since few previous studies were found in these areas, particularly in the Chinese context.

There were also several practical implications of the findings from the Fellowship. Firstly, the overall findings of the effectiveness of the SHG for the rehabilitation of former psychiatric patients in the Fellowship support the Government's rehabilitation policy in the use of informal care and self-help organizations, as stated in the 1990 Social Welfare White Paper and the 1992 Green paper on Rehabilitation Policies and Services. With evidence and recognition of the contribution of SHGs, the government should continue to provide support and development of the self-help organizations. As suggested by Mok (2001), one way to support is to establish self-help clearinghouses to maximize self-help resources and to coordinate them systematically and efficiently.

Secondly, in social work practice, theorists are arguing for the role of spirituality in psychiatric rehabilitation. This holistic care program provides some support for the importance of spiritual intervention in psychiatric rehabilitation. All findings in LUK and Shek (2006a; 2006b; 2008; 2011) support the previous studies that religion or spirituality is a factor affecting one's positive changes in terms of having more meaning of life and more hope (Kaplan et al., 1997; Pargament & Park, 1995; Saudia et al., 1991). Furthermore, these studies support the consistent findings that the positive functions of religion could help people cope with life stresses such as having an illness (Fitchett et al., 1997; Koenig et al., 1998; Schumaker, 1992; Sullivan, 1993).

Finally, based on the findings in these studies, with the modification of the holistic care program of the Fellowship, a holistic care model for psychiatric rehabilitation was developed for practice. The proposed model for practice is attached in Appendix 5. This model can be adopted by other psychiatric rehabilitation organizations for practice.

Reflection on Holistic Care

As healthcare professionals, we are all committed to provide a high quality of care to our clients. Holistic care is undoubtedly believed to be an essence of high quality professional care. Regarding the content of holistic care, there is no controversial issue in the provision of physical care since they are easily to be observed and measured such as an increase of body weight, the absence of the physical symptoms after a course of antibiotics, etc. However, there is a controversy about the psychological and spiritual care of a person. Is there a "spiritual dimension"? Is it possible that the so-called spiritual dimension is in fact a psychological dimension?

As discussed in Chapter 2, a man is viewed as a whole person consisting of different parts of his own being. However, they must not be regarded as separate or separable parts that make up what man is. It is because they are interrelated and interdependent, one component cannot be more important than the other and in fact, one cannot exist without the other. In the same vein, it is proposed by Benner (1998) not to separate the psychological and spiritual aspects of a person into two dimensions but view them as one dimension, the "psycho-spirituality". He suggested that it is difficult to separate the psychological and spiritual dimension of a person who operates as a whole being to think, act, and experience. Nevertheless, treating a person as a whole being that is integral and cannot be separated, we can still view him from different perspectives such as the physical, psychological, social, and spiritual dimensions.

For descriptive purposes, the viewing of a person from different dimensions, the psychological and spiritual dimensions, can be differentiated in the following perspectives. According to their contents, the psychological dimension is related to the mental process and its effects on behavior which are more general in nature such as instincts, drives, perceptions, emotions, etc. (Hilgard & Atkinson, 2000). Whereas in the spiritual dimension, it is related to the aspect of the underlying dimension of consciousness or the moral aspect of the soul which is specific in nature in terms of "meaning and purpose of life", the "ultimate values/reality" and "union with the super-power or God" (Canda, 1988b; Joseph, 1987; O'Brien, 1982). Regarding the boundary or domain, the psychological dimension refers to the interaction within the human being that possesses only a horizontal component. On the other hand, the spiritual dimension refers to the interaction within the human being and between the human being and the super-power that possesses both a horizontal and a vertical component (Carson, 1989; Ellison, 1983). With respect to the target of studying, the study samples of the psychological and spiritual dimensions are different. Study on the psychological dimension can use animals and human subjects, however, only human subjects can be used for study on spiritual dimension since human subjects have moral sense, understanding of virtues, and the conception of God. Virtues such as forgiveness, love, hope, humility, gratitude, self-control, and wisdom appear as highly prized elements of human nature in various religious belief systems (Emmons & Paloutzian, 2003). Several of these virtues were appraised in a special issue of the Journal of Social and Clinical Psychology and their links to physical and psychological well-being were also highlighted (McCullough & Snyder, 2000). Finally, with reference to the study of the time period, the psychological dimension focuses within one's life span, that is, from the cradle to the grave. However, the spiritual dimension will exceed one's life before birth or after death. Based on the famous western philosophers, Aristotle and the theologian, St. Thomas, it is well accepted in the western culture that the human soul, the immaterial part of a person is a substance, which is immortal and can exist independently. Therefore, when the human body, the material part of a person dies, the soul still exists (Yang, 1972). Many clinicians, especially those with a religious background, advocate that there is a spiritual dimension of a person and indicates that the spirit expresses itself through the physical and psychological dimensions of one's life but it is neither physical nor psychological (e.g., Thompson, 1984; Tournier, 1954). Furthermore, there are also research studies on the survival of consciousness after physical death which support the real existence of a spirit world that was once assumed but may now be embraced beyond reasonable doubt (Dalzell, 2002; Gauld, 1984; Martin & Romanowski, 1998; Radin, 1997; Schwartz, Simmon, & Linda, 2002). A summary of their differences is illustrated in Table 3.

Table 3. The differences between psychological and spiritual dimensions

Different Perspectives	Psychological Dimension	Spiritual Dimension
Content	Mental process and behavior	Meaning and purpose of life, ultimate values/reality, union with super-power
Boundary	Within human (horizontal)	Within and outside human (horizontal and vertical)
Study samples	Animals and human subjects	Human subjects only
Study time period	Limited within one's life span	Exceeded to life before birth or after death

As suggested by Tillich (1951), a theologian, psychologists from a psychological point of view look into how the human exists, whereas theologists from a spiritual or religious view try to understand the meaning of human existence. They both try to understand the human being from different perspectives. However, both disciplines are interrelated. Echoed by Emmons (1999), a psychologist, psychology and theology ought to be natural allies, as both are concerned, ultimately, with what it means to be a human being.

Furthermore, there are overlapping areas in both the psychological and spiritual dimensions. For example, when one searches for the meaning and purpose of life, he/she still has to think and act, which are the key areas in the psychological dimension. In other words, the spiritual dimension can also be viewed as part of the psychological dimension. Though, there is an overlapping of areas in the psychological and spiritual dimension and they are difficult to be clearly defined, there are evidences of increasing awareness of the importance of holistic care, especially in the area of spiritual dimension (Aldridge, 1993; Anderson & Young, 1988; Bergin & Jensen, 1990; Collitan, 1981). There are also increasing evidences showing the importance and effectiveness of spiritual intervention in one's health. The holistic care program provided by the Fellowship is one of the examples.

Though the definition of health in the World Health Organization (WHO) remains unchanged since 1946, which is "a state of complete physical, mental, and social well-being and not merely the absence of disease or infirmary", it is acknowledged that the spiritual dimension of health is increasingly recognized (WHO, 1998). In the structure of the quality of life scale "WHOQOL-100" developed by WHO, one of the six broad domains of the quality of life was spirituality/religion/personal beliefs, which demonstrated the importance of the spiritual dimension in one's quality of life. The other domains were physical health, psychological, level of independence, social relations, and environment (WHO, 1995; 1997). In the definition of palliative care in WHO, spiritual care of the patient is added, "Palliative care is an approach that improves the quality of life of patients and their families facing the problem associated with life-threatening illness, through the prevention and relief of suffering by means of early identification and impeccable assessment and treatment of pain and other problems, physical, psychosocial and spiritual" (WHO, 2003).

At present, many healthcare professionals have already recognized the need to consider spiritual issues within practices in order to provide a quality service. The "Religious or spiritual problem" has been established as a medical diagnosis that draws the attention of psychiatrists to the importance of the spiritual life of patients. It is described as "distressing experiences that involve loss or questioning of faith, problems associated with conversion to a new faith, or questioning of spiritual values that may not necessarily be related to an organized church or religious institution" (American Psychiatric Association, 1994, p.685). "Spiritual distress" has been developed as a nursing diagnosis that provides guidelines for nurses to meet the spiritual needs of their patients. It is described as "the state in which an individual or group experiences or is at risk of experiencing a disturbance in the belief or value system that provides strength, hope, and meaning" (Carpenito, 1993, p.301). Moreover, providing holistic care, including spiritual dimension, has also been seen as a professional standard in the nursing profession in Hong Kong (College of Nursing, Hong Kong, 1997).

In the U.S.A., all hospitals have to be accredited for the practice of healthcare services. It is the mandate of the "Joint Commission on Accreditation of Healthcare Organizations", the biggest accreditation organization in the U.S.A. that holistic care, including the bio-psycho-social-spiritual dimensions, must be provided to all patients admitted to hospitals (Joint Commission of Accreditation of Healthcare Organizations, 1992). In Hong Kong, though spiritual care is not a mandate in the healthcare services, the Nursing Section of the Hospital Authority has published a position statement on holistic care in which the provision of spiritual care is also emphasized (Hospital Authority, 2001). All nurses working in the hospitals in Hong Kong are encouraged to provide holistic care with the concern of the spiritual needs of the patients. In many hospitals, especially those with religious backgrounds, spiritual care has been integrated into the nursing practices in health assessment and care plan, complemented with in-service training on holistic care (e.g., Alice Ho Miu Ling Nethersole Hospital, 2002). With the increasing practice of holistic care by healthcare professionals, the attention of the spiritual dimension of a person, the education of spiritual care in both nursing and social work practice should be enhanced.

APPENDICES

APPENDIX 1: THE ORGANIZATION STRUCTURE OF CHRISTIAN OI HIP FELLOWSHIP

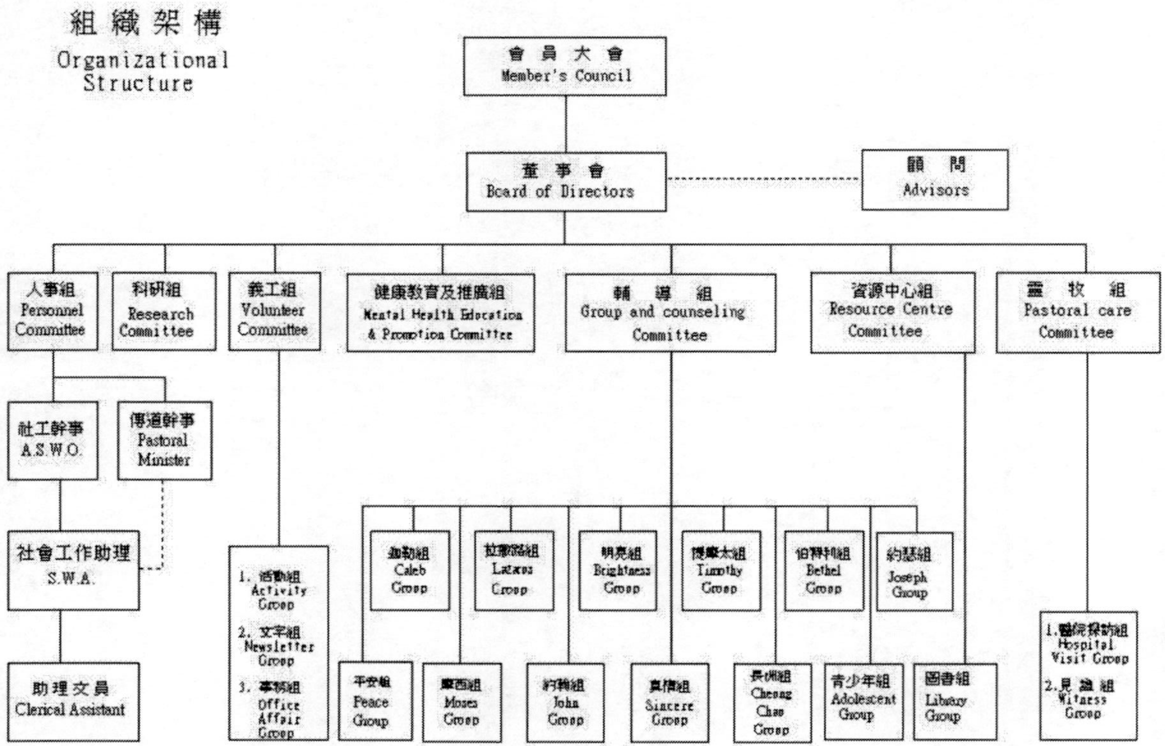

APPENDIX 2: COURSE ON "STRESS MANAGEMENT"

Aim: to study together the stress around us.

Objectives:

1. To have a comprehensive understanding about stress
2. To learn to cope with our life stress
3. To acquire a general picture of mental illness

Methods:

1. Primarily on sharing and discussion
2. Complemented with short talks, role play, psychological tests, a power-point presentation, a video, exercises, and games.

Course content:

1. What is stress?
2. Sources of stress and its effects
3. Coping with stress
4. Daily life stress
5. Stress on sex
6. Developmental stress
7. Stress on crisis
8. Occupation stress
9. Revision of coping with stress
10. Understanding of mental illness

Textbook: Collins, G. R. (1983). You can profit from stress

Course preparation

Topics	Materials	References
What is stress?	Discussion topics	Chapter 1
Sources of stress and its effects	Questionnaire on Life Changing Unit Discussion topics	Chapter 2 & 3
Coping with stress	Power-point presentation	Chapter 4
Daily life stress	Questionnaire on time spending per week	Chapter 5
Stress on sex	Q&A competition Cases for discussion Video clip Small gifts	Chapter 7 References from Hong Kong Family Planning Association
Developmental stress	Video clip	Chapter 8 References from Health education bureau
Stress on crisis	Cases for discussion	Chapter 9
Occupation stress	Questionnaire on job stress Cases for discussion	Chapter 11
Revision of coping with stress	Relaxation exercises	Chapter 12 & 13
Understanding of mental illness	Video clip	

Session Outline: What is stress?

Objectives:

1. To understand the concept of stress
2. To learn about the commonness and types of stress

Outline:

Headings	Content	Responsible person	Means	Time
Introduction	Warm up exercises	Leader	Game	15 min
Main theme	Defining stress What is stress? Can it be avoided? Is it good or bad? List what stresses you have at present?	Members	Sharing	30 min
	Definition of stress, its commonness and types	Leader	Mini – Lecture	10 min
Conclusion	Key learning points	Leader	Wrap up	5 min

Learning points:

1. Stress is difficult to define.
2. Stress is unavoidable.
3. Stress can be good or bad depending how we cope with it.
4. There are different types of stress affecting our life.

Appendix 3: Common Topics in Mutual Help Group Meetings

Physical

How to build up a good physical health?
How to manage money?
How to manage desire?
How to manage sexual drive?
How to manage time?
Facing difficulties during rehabilitation
Know more about mental illness.
Know more about psychiatric drugs
How to fight with psychiatric signs and symptoms?
How to differentiate hallucination and God's voice?
How to manage insomnia?
How to prevent relapse?
How to manage suicidal tendency?
How to communicate with your doctor?
What are the patient rights?

Mental

Managing influences from our childhood.
How to recover from psychological hurts/wounds?
Who are you? Do you understand yourself?
How to love oneself?
How to develop sense of achievement?
How to build up self confidence
How to enhance our will power?
How to manage fear?
How to manage guilty feelings?
How to face loneliness?
How to face singleness?
How to face 1997, the changing of sovereignty to PRC? (How to face change?)
How to manage emotion?
How do deal with anxiety?
How to face frustration?

How to overcome inferiority?
How to be concentrated?
How to manage anger?
How to maintain a healthy life?
How to enjoy life?

Social

How to face someone you dislike?
Learning how to give and take.
The act of caring – how to show concern for others
How to be active in developing relationship with others?
How to build up a harmonious family?
Our attitudes toward work.
How to look for a job?
How to adapt to the working environment?
How to work with our colleagues?
How to maintain a stable job?
How to courtship and develop intimate relationship with other sex?
How to maintain a marriage?

Spiritual

Why do I have to suffer? The meaning of suffering.
The art of life.
Do I have value?
What is my life goal?
How to face sins?
What is faith?
Faith and miracles.
How to understand God's will?
How to do that I was saved?
What is the right attitude toward listening God's word?
How to pray?
How to be a good Christian?
How to be a good steward?
The integration of one's beliefs and living.
How to be involved in the church life?
What is meaning for donation in church?
How to share the gospel?
How to differentiate mental illness and demon possession

Others

Sharing and praying
Outings and Picnics
Sport and recreational activities
Birthday celebration
Hiking
Movie appreciation
Festival celebration
Hymns singing
Hospital visit
Family visit
Half-way house visit
Caroling
Day or overnight retreat
Annual general meeting
Local and overseas tour

Session Outline: How to face someone you dislike

Objectives:

1. To understand the characteristics of a person whom one dislikes.
2. To learn about ways of the appropriate management of a person whom one dislikes.

Outline:

Headings	Content	Responsible person	Means	Time
Introduction	Briefing about the topic	Leader	Sharing	5 min
Main theme	Questions for sharing 1. At present, is there anyone whom you dislike? Who are they? 2. What make you dislike them? 3. How do you manage them? Present by members and a short summary made by leader	Members Leader	Sharing (dyad) (group)	10 min 20 min 10 min
Conclusion	key learning points	Leader	Mini-lecture	15 min

Learning points:

1. Avoid contact with people you dislike if possible.
2. Try to accept them
   - Look for their merits
   - Share with others
3. Manage one's emotion toward people you dislike
   - Doing exercises
   - Listening to music
   - Singing
   - Doing relaxation exercises
4. Rationally analyze to find the source of the problem

Session Outline:

How to look for a suitable job

Objectives:

1. To understand one's characters and abilities
2. To learn about the job expectation
3. To match one one's characters and abilities with the job expectation

Outline:

Headings	Content	Responsible person	Means	Time
Introduction	Briefing about the topic Game: simple personality test: (ability and interest) Source: Labor Department	Leader	Sharing	15 min
Main theme	Questions for sharing: 1. How much do you know your own characters and abilities? 2. Difficulties in looking for a job. 3. What do you expect to your job? Present by members and a short summary made by leader	Members Leader	Sharing (dyad) (group)	10 min 25 min
Conclusion	key learning points	Leader	Mini-lecture	10 min

Learning points:

1. Understand own character and abilities
2. Know the expectation of the job
3. Look for a job matched with one's character and abilities
4. Avoid over-rating or under-rating of the job requirement

Session Outline:

How to develop interpersonal relationship at work

Objectives:

1. To understand behaviors affecting relationship at work
2. To share the difficulties in developing good interpersonal relationship
3. To know the ways to develop good interpersonal relationship at work

Outline:

Headings	Content	Responsible person	Means	Time
Introduction	Briefing about the topic	Leader	Sharing	5 min
Main theme	Questions for sharing:	Members	Sharing (dyad)	
	1. What are the appropriate and inappropriate behaviors affecting interpersonal relationship at work?			10 min
	2. Difficulties in developing good interpersonal relationship at work.		(4 in a group)	10 min
	3. Ways for good relationship.		(4 in a group)	10 min
	Present by members and a short summary by leader	Leader		10 min
Conclusion	key learning points	Leader	Mini-lecture	15 min

Learning points:

1. Be aware of appropriate (e.g., friendly, mutual respect, cooperation, sincerity, appreciation, willing to help etc.) and inappropriate (e.g.,

placate, impoliteness, gossips, irresponsibility etc.) behaviors affecting interpersonal relationship at work

2. Difficulties: slow work efficiency, passive, unexpressive, unfriendly supervisor
3. Ways: passive/unexpressive – social skill training
   Work efficiency – find out the cause, set priority, enhance training, ask for help, if affected by drugs, seek for doctor's help.
   Unfriendly supervisor – know his/her expectation, patience, enhance communication, show understanding, do you best.

Session Outline:

How to face singleness

Objectives:

1. To understand own view on singleness
2. To share possible stress from singleness
3. To learn ways to face singleness

Outline:

Headings	Content	Responsible person	Means	Time
Introduction	Briefing about the topic	Leader	Sharing	5 min
Main theme	Questions for sharing 1 How much do you feel your present life as singleness i) Most enjoyable things ii) Most unbearable things 2 Ways to face stress from singleness 3 Invite sharing from successful cases Sharing by members and a short summary made by leader	Members Leader	Sharing (group)	 45 min
Conclusion	key learning points	Leader	Mini-lecture	10 min

Learning points:

1. Emphases on the positive ways for managing singleness (from enjoyable things)
2. Understand personal views on marital life
3. Accept status quo and explore potential for marriage (build up oneself to prepare for partnership)

Session Outline: Positive thinking

Objectives:

1. To understand how one views incidences
2. To learn about the advantages of positive thinking
3. To be awake of the attitudes when making decision

Outline:

Headings	Content	Responsible person	Means	Time
Introduction	To differentiate the positive thinking among different wordings	Leader	Game	5 min
Main theme	1. Definition of positive thinking & its advantages	Leader	Lecture	5 min
	2. Illustration: "water in the desert" Members are asked whether i) Glad to have water or ii) Worry no water soon	Leader	Game	10 min
	3. A case of young age cancer i) Positive – managing ii) Negative – avoidance	Members	Video Case discussion	30 min
Conclusion	key learning points	Leader	Mini-lecture	10 min

Learning points:

1. It is nature to have obstacles and difficulties in life
2. Try to clarify our thoughts and emotion attached

3. To understand the whole picture of the event on both the positive and negative aspects
4. To accept the possible negative outcomes but looking forward to the positive ones

Session Outline: How to live an enriching life

Objectives:

1. To reflect on one's present life
2. To understand what an enriching is
3. To learn how to live an enriching life

Outline:

Headings	Content	Responsible person	Means	Time
Introduction	To draw a picture to express one's present life, then sharing by dyad Or to indicate the degree of life enrichment from 0 no enrichment to 10 full of enrichment. Then invite members for sharing	Leader	Drawing	25 min
Main theme	1. What is your perception of an enriching life 2. Difficulties and management	members	sharing	25 min
Conclusion	key learning points	Leader	Mini-lecture	10 min

Learning points:

1. Know your abilities and potentials
2. Live according to one's endowment
3. Fulfill one social roles in the society as a responsible citizen

Session Outline: How to prevent relapse

Objectives:

1. To enhance understanding of one's illness
2. To learn overcoming difficulties of long-term drug treatment
3. To improve communication with case medical officer

Outline:

Headings	Content	Responsible person	Means	Time
Introduction	Briefing about the topic	Leader	Sharing	5 min
Main theme	1. Ways to enhance understanding of one's illness	Members	Sharing (Dyad)	10 min
	2. Difficulties of long-term drug treatment and ways for maintenance	Members	Sharing (4 in a group)	10 min
	3. Effective communication with case medical officer	Members	Sharing (4 in a group)	10 min
	Sharing by members and a short summary made by leader on each sub-theme	Leader		15 min
Conclusion	key learning points	Leader	Mini-lecture	10 min

Learning points:

1. Get all information from healthcare professionals, family members, friends, and other ex-patients and sensitive to one's bodily changes.
2. Understand the effects and side effects of drug and communicate with case medical officer for drug adjustment if necessary.
3. Maintain steady follow up and feedback present condition to case medical officer.

Session Outline: How to adapt to a new working environment

Objectives:

1. To know the potential problems on changing to a new environment
2. To learn the preparation for a new job

Outline:

Headings	Content	Responsible person	Means	Time
Introduction	Briefing about the topic	Leader	Sharing	5 min
Main theme	Questions for sharing 1. Potential problems for a new work environment 2. Possible solutions in facing the problems	Members	Sharing (dyad)	10 min
	3. Preparation for a new job	Leader	(group)	25 min
	Present by members and a short summary made by leader	Leader		10 min
Conclusion	key learning points	Leader	Mini-lecture	10 min

Learning points:

1. Data collection before the date of working
2. Be aware of personal stress
3. Maintain sufficient rest before taking up the new job
4. Ask for support in prayer and sharing in reducing stress

Session Outline: exploring the issue of suffering

Objectives:

1. To reflect one's view on suffering
2. To learn facing suffering in a positive way
3. To know the ways on supporting other in suffering

Outline:

Headings	Content	Responsible person	Means	Time
Introduction	Briefing about the topic	Leader	Sharing	5 min
Main theme	Questions for sharing 1. Recall an incidence of suffering 2. Explore any meaning or implication of that incidence 3. How to face suffering in a positive way? 4. How to support a loved one in facing suffering? Sharing by members and a short summary made by leader on each sub-theme	Members Members Leader	Sharing (4 in a group) Sharing in a group	15 min 15 min 15 min
Conclusion	key learning points	Leader	Mini-lecture	10 min

Learning points:

1. Many causes lead to suffering, may not have a definite answer
2. Having suffering is not an unusual life event
3. To be prepared to face suffering in one's life time
4. Having a good relationship with God is a spiritual resource in facing life crisis

APPENDIX 4: THE GROUP INTERVENTION MODEL OF THE FELLOWSHIP

Model of the Mutual Support Group (Christian Oi Hip Fellowship)

Objectives \ Stages of development	Initial Stage (app. 6 months)	Development Stage (app. One and half year)	Maturity Stage (app.2-5 years)	Self-Sustaining Stage (as long as it can be)
Develop self awareness	X----------------	----------------------------	--------------------	---------------------------→
Promote mutual understanding	X----------------	--------------------------X		
mutual acceptance	X----------------	--------------------------X		
mutual trust	X----------------	--------------------------X		
Develop group cohesiveness	X ----------------	--------------------------X		
Enhance group cohesiveness			X----------------X	
Identify potential group leader		X-------------------------X		
Develop group leader			X--------------- X	
Train group leader			X------------------	---------------------------→
Support group leader				X--------------------------→
Role of Group Counselor	Leader, facilitator.	Leader, facilitator.	Facilitator, advisor.	Advisor, overseer.
Group Program Content: (Manual prepared) Structure: Theme & Sharing (Biweekly alternatively)	Stress Management	Initiated by members and coordinated by group counselor	Initiated and coordinated by group committee elected by themselves	

APPENDIX 5: THE HOLISTIC CARE MODEL FOR PSYCHIATRIC REHABILITATION

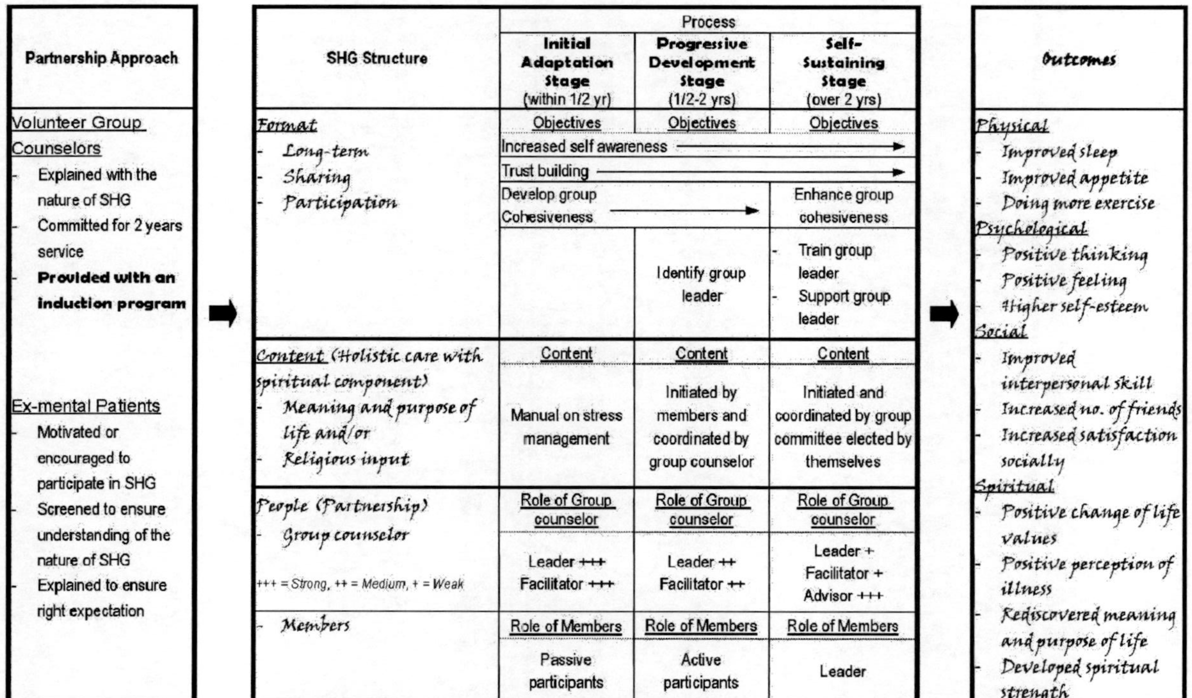

Remarks: *Features based on the findings of the three studies* **Modification from the holistic care program of the Fellowship**

REFERENCES

Abbot, N. C., Harkness, E. F., Stevinson, C., Marshall, F. P., Conn, D. A, & Ernst, E. (2001). Spiritual healing as a therapy for chronic pain: A randomized, clinical trial. *Pain, 91,* 79-89.

Abramowitz, L. (1993). Prayer as therapy among the frail Jewish elderly. *Journal of Gerontological Social Work, 19*(3/4), 69-75.

Action Committee Against Narcotics. (2002). *The Hong Kong Narcotics Report 2002.* Hong Kong: Narcotics Division, Government of HKSAR.

Adams, R. (1990). *Self-help, social work and empowerment.* London: Macmillan.

Ai, A. (2000). Spiritual well-being, population aging, and a need for improving practice with the elderly: A psychosocial account. *Social Thought, 19*(3), 1-21.

Alcoholics Anonymous (1955). New York: *Alcoholics Anonymous,* 569.

Aldridge, D. (1993). Is there evidence for spiritual healing? ADVANCES, *The Journal of Mind-Body Health, 9*(4), 4-21.

Alford, G. S., Koehler, R. A., & Leonard, J. (1991). Alcoholics Anonymous: Narcotics Anonymous model inpatient treatment of chemically-dependent adolescents: A two year outcome study. *Journal of Studies on Alcohol, 52,* 118-126.

Alice Ho Miu Ling Nethersole Hospital. (2001, March). Holistic care fortnight, *Hospital Newsletter,17.*

Alice Ho Miu Ling Nethersole Hospital. (2002). *Annual Report,* 2001-2002, 64.

Allen, C.E. (1991a). An analysis of the pragmatic consequences of holism for nursing. *Western Journal of Nursing Research, 13,* 256-272.

Allen, C.E. (1991b). Holistic concepts and the professionalization of public health nursing. *Public Health Nursing, 8,* 74-80.

Allport, G. W & Ross, J. M. (1967). Personal religious orientation and prejudice. *Journal of Personality and Social Psychology, 5,* 432-443.

American Holistic Nursing Association. (2012). The past, present and future. Retrieved 25/6/2012 from website: http://www.ahna.org/

American Psychiatric Association. (APA) (1994). *Diagnostic and statistical manual of mental disorder* (4th ed). Washington, DC: Author.

Anandarajah, G., & Hight, E. (2001). Spirituality and medical practice: using the HOPE questions as a practical tool for spiritual assessment. *American Family Physician, 63*(1), 81-89.

Anderson, R.G. & Young, J.L. (1988). The religious component of acute hospital treatment. *Hospital and Community Psychiatry, 39(5),* 528-55.

Argyle, M., & Beit-Hallahmi, B. (1975). *The social psychology of religion.* London: Routledge & Kegan Paul. (Original work published 1958).

Assagioli, R. (1971). *Psychosynthesis: A manual of principles and techniques.* New York: Viking. (Original work published 1965)

Assagioli, R. (1993). *Transpersonal development: The dimension beyond psychosynthesis.* San Franciso: Aquarian.

Astin, J. A., Harkness, E., & Ernst, E. (2000). The efficacy of distant healing: a systematic review of randomized trials. *Annals of Internal Medicine, 132*(11), 903-910.

Aston, J. (1984, May). The power of the will. *Nursing Times, 80* (2).

Azhart, M. A., Varma, S. L., & Dharap, A. S. (1994). Religious psychotherapy in anxiety disorder patients. *Acta Psychiatric Scandinavica, 90,* 1-3.

Baier, C. J., & Wright, B. R. E. (2001). "If you love me, keep my commandments": A meta-analysis of the effect of religion on crime. *Journal of Research in Crime & Delinquency, 38*(1), 3-21.

Bankoff, E. A. (1979). Widow groups as an alternative to informal social support. In M. A. Lieberman, & L. D. Borman (Eds.), *Self-help groups for coping with crisis* (pp. 189-193). San Farncisco: Jossey Bass.

Bardill, D.R. (1976). The making of a person. *Social Thought,* 15-26.

Barnum, B.S. (1995, Spring). Spirituality in Nursing. *Nursing Leadership Forum, 1*(1), 24-30.

Batson, C. D., & Ventis, W. L. (1982). *The religious experience.* New York: Oxford University Press.

Becker, T., Thornicroft, G., Leese, M., McCrone, P, Johnson, S., Albert, M., & Turner, D. (1997). Social networks and service use among representatives cases of psychosis in south London. *British Journal of Psychiatry, 171,* 15-19.

Bednur, R. L. & Kaul, T. J. (1978). Experiential groups research: Current perspectives. In S.L. Garfield & A. E. Bergin (eds.) *Handbook of psychotherapy and behavior change* (pp. 769-826). New York: Wiley.

Belknap, M., Blau, R., & Grossman, R. (eds) (1979). *Case studies and methods in humanistic medicine.* San Francisco: Institute for the Study of Humanistic Medicine, p.18.

Belton, W.J. (1994). *Mutual aid – support groups: A study of the roles social workers assume with this informal system of care.* USA: Bell & Howell Company.

Benner, D. G. (1988). *Psychotherapy and the spiritual quest.* Grand Rapids, Mich: Baker Book House.

Benner, D. G. (1998). *Care of souls.* Grand Rapids, Mich: Baker Book House.

Benson, H., Dusek, J. A., Sherwood, J. B., Lam, P., Bethea, C. F., Carpenter, W., Levitsky, S. et al.,(2006). Study of the therapeutic effects of intercessory prayer (STEP) in cardiac bypass patients: A multicenter randomized trial of uncertainty and certainty of receiving intercessory prayer, *American Heart Journal, 151*(4), 934-42.

Benson, P. L. (1992). Religion and substance use. In J. F. Schumaker (Ed.), *Religion and mental health* (pp. 211-221). New York: Oxford University Press.

Bergin, A. E. (1980). Psychotherapy and religious values. *Journal of Consulting and Clinical Psychology, 48,* 95-105.

Bergin, A. E. (1983). Religiosity and mental health: a critical reevaluation meta-analysis. *Professional Psychology: Research and Practice, 14,* 170-184.

Bergin, A. E. (1985). Values and psychotherapy. In D. G. Benner (Ed.), *Baker Encyclopedia of Psychology* (pp. 1191-1194). Grand Rapids, MI: Baker Book House.

Bergin, A. E. (1991). Values and religious issues in psychotherapy and mental health. *American Psychologist, 46,* 4, 394-403.

Bergin, A. E., & Jensen, J. P. (1990). Religiosity of psychotherapists: A national survey. *Psychotherapy, 27,* 3-7.

Bergin, A. E., Stinchfield, R. D., Gaskin, T. A., Master, K. S., & Sullivan, C. E. (1988). Religious life-styles and mental health: An exploratory study. *Journal of Counseling Psychology, 35,* 91-98.

Blattner, B. (1981). *Holistic nursing.* Englewoold Cliffs, N.J.: Prentice-Hall, Inc.

Bowler, S. (2008). The object of medicine In D. Wainwright eds. A Sociology of Health, p39. London: SAGE publication

Boyd, T. A. (1998). Spiritually sensitive assessment tools for social work practice. In B. Hugen (Ed.), *Christianity and social work: Readings on the integration of Christian faith and social work practice* (pp. 239-255). Botsford, CT: NACSW Press.

Bradshaw, A. (1994). *Breaking the lamp.* London: Scutari Press.

Brandon, D. (1976). *Zen in the art of helping.* New York: Delta/Seymour Lawrence.

Brennan, J. F. (1982). *History and systems of psychology.* Englewood Cliffs, NJ: Prentice-Hall.

Breton, M. (1989). Liberation theology, group work, and the right of the poor and oppressed to participate in the life of the community. *Social Work With Groups, 12(3),* 5-18.

Brown, G. W., & Prudo, R. (1981). Psychiatric disorder in a rural and an urban population. I: Aetiology of depression. *Psychological Medicine, 11,* 581-599.

Brown, H. P., & Peterson, J. H. (1991). Assessing spirituality in addition to treatment and follow-up: Development of the Brown-Peterson Recovery Progress Inventory (B-PRPI). *Alcoholism Treatment Quarterly, 8,* 21-50.

Brown, L. B. (1994). *Religion, personality, and mental health.* New York: Springer.

Bufford, R. (1981). *The human reflex: Behavioral psychology in Christian perspective.* San Francisco: Harper & Row.

Bullis, R. K. (1996). *Spirituality in social work practice.* Washington, DC: Taylor & Francis.

Burkhardt, M. & Nagai-Jacobson, M. (1985). Dealing with spiritual concerns at clients in the community. *Journal of Community Health Nursing, 2,* 191-198.

Byrd, R. C. (1988). Positive therapeutic effects of intercessory prayer in a coronary care unit population. *Southern Medical Journal, 81,* 826-9.

Callan, J. (1979). Holistic health or holistic hoax. *Journal of the American Medical Association, 241,* 1156

Canda, E. R. (1988a). Conceptualizing spirituality for social work: Insights from diverse perspectives. *Social Thought, 14*(1), 30-46.

Canda, E. R. (1988b). Spirituality, religious diversity, and social work practice. *Social Casework, 69*, 238-247.

Canda, E. R. (1989). Religious content in social work education: A comparative approach. *Journal of Social Work Education, 25,* 36-45.

Canda, E. R. (1991). East/West philosophical synthesis in transpersonal theory. *Journal of sociology and Social Welfare, 18(4),* 137-152.

Canda, E. R. (1997). Spirituality In Edward, R. L. (Ed.), *Encyclopedia of Social Work. Supplement* (pp. 299-309). Washing, D.C.: NASW Press.

Canda, E. R. (2002). The significance of spirituality for resilient response to chronic illness: A qualitative study of adults with cystic fibrosis. In D, Saleebey (Ed.), *The Strengths Perspective in Social Work Practice* (pp. 63-79). New York: Longman.

Canda, E. R. & Furman, L. D. (1999*). Spiritual diversity in social work practice:* The heart of helping. New York: Free press.

Canda, E. R. & Phaobtong, T. (1992). Buddhism as a support system for Southeast Asian refugees. *Social Work, 37,* 61-67

Caplan, G. (1974). *Support System and Community Mental Health.* New York: Behavioral Publications. (pp.1- 40).

Carpenito, L. J. (1983). Nursing Diagnosis: Application to clinical practice. New York: Lippincott.

Carroll, M. M. (1997). Spirituality and clinical social work: Implications of past and current perspectives. *Arete, 62*(1), 25-34.

Carroll, S. (1993). Spirituality and purpose in life in alcoholism recovery. *Journal of Studies on Alcohol, 54,* 297-301.

Carson, V.B. (1989). *Spiritual dimensions of nursing practice.* (pp. 13-20) Philadelphia: Saunders.

Cattell, J. M. (1947). The progress of psychology. In A. T. Poffenberger (Ed.), *James McKeen Cattell: Man of science. (Vol.2).*

Chamiec-Case, R. (2009). Developing a scale to measure social workers' integration of spirituality in the workplace, *Journal of Religion and Spirituality in Social Work: Social Thought, 28*:3, 284-305.

Chan, C., Chow, A., Au, T. , Leung, P., Chau, P., Chang, F., Ma, J., Cheng. B.Y., & Tam. V. (1996). *Therapeutic Groups in Medical Settings.* Resource Paper No. 25. University of Hong Kong: Department of Social Work & Social Administration.

Chan, C., Wong, D., Ho, P. Ip, F. & Tong, H. (1992). *Report of a Survey of the members of Self-help Groups for Persons with Chronic Illness in Hong Kong.* Hong Kong: University of Hong Kong, Department of Social Work & Social Administration.

Chen, C. H. (1979). The neurophysiological mechanism of acupuncture treatment in psychiatric illness: An autonomic-humoral theory. *American Journal of Chinese Medicine, 7,* 183-187.

Cherniss, C., & Cherniss, D. S. (1987). Professional involvement in self-help groups for parents of high-risk newborns. *American Journal of Community Psychology, 15,* 435-444

Chesler, M. A. (1990). The"dangers"of self-help groups: Understanding and challenging professionals'views. In T. J. Powell, *Working with self-help* (pp. 301-324). Silver Spring, MD: NASW Press.

Chesler, M. A., & Chesney, B. K. (1995). *Cancer and self-help: Bridging the troubled waters of childhood illness.* Madison, WI: University of Wisconsin Press.

Chien, W. T., Chan, S., Morrissey, J., & Thompson, D. (2005). Effectiveness of a mutual support group for families of patients with schizophrenia. *Journal of Advanced Nursing, 51*(6), 595-608.

Chien, W. T., Chan, S. W. C., Morrissey, J., & Thompson, D. (2006). Effects of a mutual support group for Chinese people with schizophrenia: 18-month follow-up. *British Journal of Psychiatry, 189,* 41-49. Doi:10.1192/bjp.bp.105.008375

Chiu, L. (2000). Lived experience of spirituality in Taiwanese women with breast cancer. *Western Journal of Nursing Research, 22,* 29-35

Chu, C. C., & Klein, H. E. (1985). Psychosocial and environmental variables in outcome of black schizophrenics. *Journal of the National Medical Association, 77,* 793-796.

Clay S (2005) *On our own, together: Peer programs for people with mental illness.* Vanderbilt University Press, Nashville.

Clinebell, H. J. (1970). The local church's contribution to positive mental health. In J. J. Clinebell (Ed.), *Community mental health: The role of church and temple.* Nashville, TN: Abingdon Press.

Cockerham, W.C. (1986). *Medical sociology.* (p. 84, 115) New Jersey: Prentice-Hall, Inc.

Cohen, J. (1989). Spiritual healing in a medical context. *Practitioner, 233*(1473), 1056-7.

College of Nursing. (1997). *Standard for psychiatric nursing practice: Standards and criteria.* Hong Kong: Hong Kong College of Nursing.

Collins, G. R. (1980). *Christian counseling.* Waco, TX: Word Press.

Collitan, M. (1981). The spiritual dimensions of nursing. In I. Beland, & J. Posses (eds.), *Clinical nursing: Pathophysiological and psychosocial approach.* New York: Macmilan.

Comstock, C. M., & Mohamoud, J. L. (1990). Professionally facilitated self-help groups: Benefits for professionals and members. In T. J. Powell

(Ed.), *Working with self help* (pp. 177-188). Silver Spring Md: NASW Press.

Conco, D. (1995). Christian patients'views of spiritual care. *Western Journal of Nursing Research, 17*(3), 266-276.

Constable, R. T. (1983). Values, religion, and social work practice. *Social Thought, 9*(4), 29-41.

Cook, T. L. (1980). Preface. In Cook, T. C. (ed.), *Spiritual well-being of the elderly*. Springfield, IL: Charles C Thomas.

Corey, G. (1990). *Theory and practice of group counseling.* (3rd Ed.), (pp.13-16). California: Cole Publishing Company.

Cortright, B. (1997). *Psychotherapy and spirit: Theory and practice in transpersonal psychotherapy.* Albany: State university of New York Press.

Coulon, L., Mok, M., Krause, K-L., & Anderson, M. (1996). The pursuit of excellence in nursing care: what does it mean? *Journal of Advanced Nursing, 24,* 817-826.

Cowley, A. S. (1993). Transpersonal social work: A theory for the 1990s. *Social Work, 38,* 527-534.

Cowley, A. S. & Derezotes, D. (1994). Transpersonal psychology and social work education. *Journal of Social Work Education, 30,* 32-41.

Cox, D. R. (1983). Religion and the welfare of immigrants. *Australian Social Work, 36*(1), 3-10.

Cox, T. (2003). Theory and exemplars of advanced practice spiritual intervention. *Complementary Therapies in Nursing & Midwifery, 9,* 30-34.

Craigie, F. C., Larson, D. B. & Liu, I. Y. (1990). References to religion in the Journal of Family Practice: dimensions and valence of spirituality. *Journal of Family Practice, 30,* 477-480.

Crawford, R. (1977). You are dangerous to your health: The ideology and politics of victim blaming. *International Journal of Health Service, 7,* 663-680

Dadich, A. (2007). Is spirituality important to young people in recovery? Insights from participants of Self-Help Support Group, *Southern Medical Journal, 100*(4), 422-425.

Dalzell, G.(2002). *Messages: Evidence for life after death.* Novato: New World Library.

Davies, P. (1992). *The mind of god: The scientific basis for a rational world.* New York: Simon & Schuster.

Delgado, M. (1996). Religion as a caregiving system for Puerto Rican elders with functional disabilities. *Journal of Gerontological Social Work, 26*(3/4), 129-44.

Dennis, P. (1991). Components of spiritual nursing care from the nurses' perspective. *Journal of Holistic Nursing, 9*(1), 27-42.

Derezotes, D. S., & Evans, K. E. (1995). Spirituality and religiosity in practice: In-depth interviews of social work practitioners. *Social Thought, 18*(1), 39-56.

Dittes, J. E. (1969). The psychology of religion. In G. Lindzey & E, Aronson (Eds.), *The handbook of social psychology (vol.5)* (pp. 602-659). Reading, MA: Addison-wesley.

Dolgoff, R., & Feldstein, D. (1980). *Understanding social welfare*. NY: Harper & Row.

Donahue, M. J., & Benson, P. L. (1995). Religion and the well-being of adolescents. *Journal of Social Issues, 51,* 145-160.

Donahue, M. J.(1985). Intrinsic and extrinsic religiousness: Review and meta-analysis. *Journal of Personality and Social Psychology, 48,* 400-419.

Doran, R. (1979). Jungian psychology and Christian spiritually: III. *Review for Religions, 38,* 857-66.

Douglas, J.D., Bruce, F.F., Packer, J.I., Hillyer, N., Guthrie, D., Millard, A.R. & Wiseman, D.J. (1984). *New Bible Dictionary* (2nd ed.) (pp. 145, 379, 731, 1135-37). Wheaton, Illinois: Tyndale House Publishers, Inc.,

DuBos, R. (1959). *The Mirage of Health.* New York: Harper and Row.

DuBos, R. (1969). *Man, medicine, and environment.* New York: Mentor.

Dull, V. T. & Skokan, L. A. (1995). A cognitive model of religion's influence on health. In R. F. Paloutzian & L. A. Kirkpaatrick (eds.), *Journal of Social Issues, 51*(2), (pp. 49-62).

Durkheim, E. (1961). *The elementary forms of religious life.* New York: Collier.

Edlin, G., & Golanty, E. (1992). *Health and wellness: A holistic approach* (4th eds). Boston, Mass. : Jones and Bartlett.

Eisenberg, D., David, R. B., Ettner, S. L., et al., (1998). Trends in alternative medicine use in the United States; 1990-1997. *Journal of the American Medical Association, 280*(18), 1569-1575.

Ellis, A. (1980). Psychotherapy and atheistic values: A response to A.E. Bergin's "Psychotherapy and Religious Issues."*Journal of Consulting and Clinical Psychology, 48,* 635-39.

Ellis, A. (1989). Dangers of transpersonal psychology: A reply to Ken Wilber. *Journal of Counseling and Development, 67,* 336-337.

Ellis, A., & Schoenfeld, E. (1990). Divine intervention and the treatment of chemical dependency. *Journal of Substance Abuse, 2,* 459-468.

Ellison, C. G. (1992). Are religious people nice? Evidence from the national survey of Black Americans. *Social Forces, 71(*2), 411-430.

Ellison, C. W. (1983). Spiritual well-being: Conceptualization and measurement. *Journal of Psychology and Theology, 11,* 330-340.

Emerick, R. (1990). Self-help groups for former patients: Relations with mental health professionals. *Hospital and Community Psychiatry, 42*(4), 401-407.

Emmons, R. A. (1999). The psychology of ultimate concerns: Motivation, cognition, and the psychology of ultimate concern. *International Journal of Psychology and Religion. 10*, 3-26.

Emmons, R. A., & Paloutzian, R. F. (2003). The psychology of religion. *Annual Review of Psychology. 54,* 377-402.

Engel, G.L. (1977). The need for a new medical model: A challenge for biomedicine. *Science, 196,* 129-136.

Ernst, E. (2006). Spiritual healing: More than meets the eye. *Journal of Pain and Symptom Management. 32*(5), 393-395.

Fergusson, A. (1995). Alternative medicine. In M.D. Beer, *Christian choices in healthcare* (pp. 236-243). London: Inter-Varsity Press..

Fischer, K. (1985). *Winter grace.* New York: Paulist Press.

Fish, S. & Shelly, J.A. (1978). *Spiritual care: The nurse's role.* Downers Grove, IL: InterVarsity Press.

Fitchett, G., Burton, L. A., & Sivan, A. B. (1997). The religious needs and resources of psychiatric patients. *Journal of Nervous and Mental Disease, 185,* 320-326.

Forbes, M.A. (2000). Complementary and alternative therapies in nursing and health care. In J. Zerwekh & J.C. Claborn (eds.), *Nursing today: Transition and trend* (pp. 301-318). Philadelphia: Saunders.

Forsyth, J. (1997). *Faith and human transformation: A dialogue between psychology and theology* (p.181). Lanham, Md: University Press of America.

Frankl, V. (1963). *Man's search for meaning: An introduction to logotherapy.* New York: Simon and Schuster.

Freud, S. (1910). Leonardo Da Vinci. In *The standard edition of the complete psychological works of Sigmund Freud,* trans. and ed. J. Strachey, vol. 11. London: Hogarth.

Freud, S. (1913).Totem and taboo. In *The standard edition of the complete psychological works of Sigmund Freud,* trans. and ed. J. Strachey, vol. 13. London: Hogarth.

Freud, S. (1966).Obsessive actions and religious practices. In *The standard edition of the complete psychological works of Sigmund Freud,* trans. and ed. J. Strachey, vol. 1. London: Hogarth.

Fromm, E. (1950). *Psychoanalysis and religion.* New Haven, CT: Yale University Press.

Fuller, A. R. (1994). *Psychology and religion: Eight points of view.* Maryland: Rowman and Littlefield Publishers, Inc.

Fuller, R.C. (1996). Holistic health practices. In Peter H. Van Ness (ed.), *Spirituality and the secular quest.* New York: Crossroad Publishing Co.

Galinsky, M. J., & Schopler, J. H. (1994). Negative experiences in support groups. *Social Work in Health Care, 20*(1), 77-95.

Garb, J. R., & Stunkard, A. (1974). Effectiveness of a self-help group in obesity control: Further assessment. *Archives of International Medicine, 134,* 716-26.

Gartner, A., & Riessman, F. (1977). *Self-help in the human services.* San Francisco: Jossey. Bass, Inc.

Gartner, A., & Riessman, F. (1982) Self-help and mental health. *Hospital and Community Psychiatry, 33* (8), 631-35.

Gartner, A. & Riessman, F. (1984). *The Self-help revolution.* (pp. 17-23, 243-248). New York: Human Sciences Press.

Gartner, J., Larson, D. B., & Allen, G. D. (1991). Religious commitment and mental health: A review of empirical literature. *Journal of Psychology and Theology, 19,* 6-25.

Gauld, A. (1984). *Mediumship and survival: A century of investigations.* Chicago: Academy.

George, Y. S., Richardson, V., Lakes-Matyas, M., & Blake, F. (1989). *Saving minds: Black churches and education.* Washington, DC: American Association for the Advancement of Science.

Gordon, A., Merenstein, J. H., D'Amico, F. & Hudgens, D. (1998). The effects of therapeutic touch on patients with osteoarthritis of knee. *Journal of Family Practice. 47,* 271-7.

Gordon, J.S. (1980). The paradigm of holistic medicine. In A. Hasting, J. Fadiman, & J.S. Gordon (Eds.), *Health for the whole person* (pp. 3-25). Boulder, CO: Westview Press.

Gordon, J.S. (1982). Holistic medicine: Advances and shortcomings. *Western Journal of Medicine, 136,* 546-551.

Gordon, J.S. (1990, July). Holistic medicine and mental health practice: Toward a new synthesis. *American Journal of Orthopsychiatry, 60*(3), 357-370.

Graham, M. A., Kaiser, T., & Garrett, K. J. (1998). Naming the spiritual: The hidden dimension of helping. *Social Thought, 18*(4), 49-61.

Griffith, E. E., & Young, J. L. (1988). A cross-cultural introduction to the therapeutic aspects of Christian religious ritual. In L. Comas-Diaz, & E. E. Griffith, *Clinical guidelines in cross-cultural mental health* (pp. 69-89). New York: Wiley & Sons.

Grimsmo, A., Helgesen, G., & Borchgrevink, C. (1981), Short-term and long-term effects of lay groups on weight reduction. *British Journal of Medicine, 283,* 1093-1095.

Grof, S., & Grof, C. (1989). *Spiritual emergency: When personal transformation becomes a crisis.* Los Angeles: Tarcher.

Guo, X. F., Zhou, B., Nishimura, T., Teramukai, S., & Fukushima, M. (2008). Clinical effect of Qigong practice on essential hypertension: A meta-analysis of randomized controlled trials. *Journal of Alternative and Complementary Medicine, 14* (1), 27-37.

Guthrie, R. (1945). *A History of medicine.* London: Thomas Nelson.

Haight, W. L. (1998)."Gathering the spirit"at first Baptist church: Spirituality as a protective factor in the lives of African American children. *Social Work, 43*(3), 213-221.

Hamilton, N. G., Ponzoha, C. A., Cutler, D. L., & Weigel, R. M. (1989). Social networks and negative versus positive symptoms of schizophrenia. *Schizophrenia Bulletin, 15*(4), 625-633.

Hansen G. (1992). Religion and marital adjustment. In J. F. Schumaker (Ed.), *Religion and mental health* (pp. 189-198). New York: Oxford University Press.

Hardiman, E. R., & Segal, S. P. (2003). Community membership and social networks in mental health self-help agencies. *Psychiatric Rehabilitation Journal, 27*(1), 25-33.

Harris, W. S., Gowda, M, Kolb, J. W., Strychacs, C. P., Vacek, J. L., Jones, P. G., Forker, A., O'Keefe, J. H. & McCallister, B. D. (1999). A randomised controlled trial of the effects of remote, intercessory prayer on outcomes in patients admitted to the coronary care unit. *Archive of Internal Medicine. 159*, 2273-8.

Hawley, G. & Irurita, V. (1998). Seeking comfort through prayer. *International Journal of Nursing Practice, 4*, 9-18.

Hemphill-Pearson, B.J. & Hunter, M. (1997). Holism in mental health practice. *Occupational Therapy in Mental Health,13*(2), 35-49.

Henry, S., & Robinson, D. (1978). Understanding Alcoholics Anonymous. *Lancet, 1,* 372-375.

Hepworth, D. & Larsen, J. A. (1986). *Direct social work practice: Theory and skills* (p.549). Homewood, IL: Dorsey Press,

Hiatt, J. (1986). Spirituality, medicine, and healing. *Southern Medical Journal, 79*(6), 736-43.

Highfield, M. F., & Cason, C. (1983). Spiritual needs of patients: Are they recognized? *Cancer Nursing, 6*, 187-192

Hilgard, E.R., Atkinson, R. L., & Alkinson, R.C. (1979). *Introduction to psychology* (p. 8). New York: Harcourt Brace Jovanovich.

Hilgard, E.R. & Atkinson, R. L. (2000). *Hilgard's introduction to psychology*. Fort worth, London: Harcourt Brace College Publishers.

Hinrichsen, G.A., Revenson, T.A. & Shinn, M. (1985). Does self-help help? An empirical investigation of scoliosis peer support groups. *Journal of Social Issues, 41,* 65-87.

Hinshaw, D. B. (2002). The spiritual needs of the dying patient._*Journal of American College of Surgeon, 195*(4), 565-568.

Hodge, D. R. (1998). Welfare reform and religious providers: An examination of the new paradigm. *Social Work & Christianity, 25*(3), 24-48.

Hodge, D. R. (2000a). Spirituality: Towards a theoretical framework. *Social Thought, 19*(4), 1-20.

Hodge, D. R. (2000b). Do faith-based providers respect client autonomy? A comparison of client and staff perceptions in faith-based and secular residential treatment programs. *Social Thought, 19*(3), 39-57.

Hodge, D. R. (2001). Spiritual assessment: A review of major qualitative methods and a new framework for assessing spirituality. *Social Work, 46*(3), 203-214.

Hodge, D. R., & Horvath, V. E. (2011). Spiritual needs in health care settings: A qualitative meta-synthesis of clients' perspectives. 56(4), 306-316.

Holland, T. (1989, Winter). Values, faith, and professional practice. *Social Thought,* 15(1), 28-40.

Hollywell, C., & Walker, J. (2008). Private prayer as a suitable intervention for hospitalized patients: A critical review of the literature. *Journal of Clinical Nursing, 18,* 637-651.

Hong Kong Government (1991). *Social welfare into the 90's and beyond.* Hong Kong: The Government Printer.

Hong Kong Government (1992). *Green paper on rehabilitation – Equal opportunities and full participation: A better tomorrow for all.* Hong Kong: Government Printer.

Hong Kong Government (1993). *Towards better health – A consultation document.* Hong Kong: The Government Printer.

Hong Kong Government (1995). *White paper on rehabilitation – equal opportunities and full participation: A better tomorrow for all.* Hong Kong: The Government Printer.

Hong Kong Government (1998). *The five year plan for social welfare development in Hong Kong-review 1998.* Hong Kong: Government Printer

Hong Kong Government (1999). *Hong Kong rehabilitation program plan: Towards a new rehabilitation era* (p.174). Rehabilitation Division, Health and Welfare Bureau. Government Secretariat.

Hospital Authority. (2001). *Position statement on holistic nursing.* Nursing Section, Hong Kong: Hospital Authority.

Humphreys, K., & Noke, J.M. (1997). The influence of post treatment mutual help group participation on the friendship networks of substance abuse patients. *American Journal of Community Psychology, 25*(1), 1-16.

Iggulden, T. (1996). Career patients: Prove care system failure-long-term help inadequate, say experts. *Window, 5*(25), 10-11.

Illich, I. (1977). *Limits to medicine. London :* Pelican Books.

James, W. (1961). *The varieties of religious experience.* New York: Macmillan Collier Books. (Original work published 1902).

Johnson, M.B. (1990). The holistic paradigm in nursing: The diffusion of an innovation. *Research in Nursing & Health, 13,* 129-139.

Jones, S. L. (1988). A religious critique of behavior therapy. In W. R. Miller & J. E. Martin (Eds.), *Behavior therapy and religion-integrating spiritual and behavioral approaches to change* (pp. 139-170). Newbury Park: sage Publications.

Jones, S. L. (1994). A constructive relationship for religion with the science and profession of psychology: Perhaps the boldest model yet. *American Psychologist, 49,* 184-199.

Jorm, A. F., Christensen, H., Griffiths, K. M., & Rodgers, B. (2002). Effectiveness of complementary and self-help treatments for depression. *Medical Journal of Australia, 176*, S84-S96.

Joseph, M. (1987). The religious and spiritual aspects of clinical practice: A neglected dimension. *Social Thought, 13*(1), 12-23.

Joseph, M. (1988). Religion and social work practice. *Social Casework, 60,* 443-452.

Jung, C. (1936). Psychoanalysis and the cure of souls. In N. Read, M. Fordham, and G. Adler (eds.), *The collected works of C.G. Jung* vol. 11. Princeton: Princeton University Press.

Kaplan, M. S., Marks, G., & Mertens, S. B. (1997). Distress and coping among women with HIV infection: preliminary findings from a multiethnic sample. *American Journal of Orthopsychiatry, 67(1)*, 80-91.

Karp, D. A., & Tanarugsachock, V. (2000). Mental illness, caregiving, and emotion management. *Qualitative Health Research, 10*(1), 6-25.

Kaslof, L.J. (1978). *Wholistic dimensions in healing: A resource guide.* New York: Doubleday.

Kaslow, F., & Robison, J. A. (1996). Long-term satisfying marriages: Perceptions contributing factors. *The American Journal of Family Therapy, 24*(2), 153-170.

Katz, A.H. (1970). Self-help organization and volunteer participation in social welfare. *Social Work, 15*(1), 51-60.

Katz, A. H. (1993). *Self help in America: A social movement perspective.* New York: Twayne Publishers.

Katz, A. H. & Bender, E. I. (1976). *The strength in us: Self-help groups in the modern world.* New Viewpoints, New York: Frankin Watts.

Kehoe, N. C. (1999). A therapy group on spiritual issues for patients with chronic mental illness. *Psychiatric Services. 50*(8), 1081-1083.

Kehoe N (2007) Spirituality groups in serious mental illness. *Southern Medical Journal 100(6), 647-648.*

Kelly, E. W. Jr. (1995). *Spirituality and religion in counseling and psychotherapy*. New York: Springer.

Kennedy, J. E., Davis, R. C., & Talyor, B. G. (1998). Changes in spirituality and well-being among victims of sexual assault. *Journal for the Scientific Study of Religion, 37*(2), 322-328.

Kierkegaard, S. (1954). *Fear and trembling and the sickness unto death.* Princeton: Princeton University Press.

Kilpatrick, A.C., & Holland, T.P. (1990). Spiritual dimensions of practice. *The Clinical Supervisor, 8*(2), 125-140.

Kimble, M., McFadeen, S., Ellor, J., & Seeber, J. (1995). *Aging, spirituality, and religion*. Minneapolis: Fortress Press.

Kinsella, K. B., Anderson, R. A., & Anderson, W. T. (1996). Coping skills, strengths, and needs as perceived by adult offspring and siblings of people with mental illness: A Retrospective study. *Psychiatric Rehabilitation Journal, 20*(2), 24-32.

Klass, D. (1992). Religious aspects in the resolution of parental grief: Solace and social support. In K.I. Pargament, K.I. Maton, & R.E. Hess (Eds.), *Religion and prevention in mental health: Research, vision, and action* (pp. 156-178). New York: The Haworth Press.

Koenig, H. G. (1997). *Is religion good for your health?* New York: Haworth Press.

Koenig, H. G. (1998). *Handbook of religion and mental health.* California: Academic Press.

Koenig, H. G. (2009). Research on religion, spirituality, and mental health: A review. *Canadian Journal of Psychiatry, 54*(5), 283-291.

Koenig, H. G., Cohen, H. J., Blaer, F. H., Peiper, C., Meador, K. G., Shelp. F., Goli, V., & DiPasquale. R. (1992). Religious coping and depression among elderly, hospitalied medically ill men. *American Journal of Psychiatry, 149,* 1693-1700.

Koenig, H. G., George, L. K., & Peterson, B. L. (1998). Religiosity and remission from depression in medically ill older patients. *American Journal of Psychiatry, 155,* 536-542.

Koenig, H. G., & Weaver, A. J. (1997). *Counseling troubled older adults: A handbook for clergy and religious caregivers.* Nashvill, TN: Abingdon Press.

Koenig, T. L., & Spano, R. N. (1998). Taoism and the strengths perspective. Social Thought, 18(2), 47-65.

Kopas, J. (1981). Jung and Assagioli in religious perspective. *Journal of Psychology and Theology, 9,* 216-23.

Koslander, T., & Arvidsson, B. (2007). Patients' conception of how the spiritual dimension is addressed in mental health care: a qualitative study. *Journal of Advanced Nursing, 57*(6), 597-604.

Krause, N. (1995). Religiostiy and self-esteem among older adults. *Journal of Geronotology, 50*, 236-246

Krieger, D. (1975). *The Therapeutic Touch* (p.13). Englewood Cliffs, N.J.:Prentice-Hall.

Krill, D. (1978). *Existential social work.* New York: Free Press.

Kropotkin, P. (1955). *Mutual aid: A factor of evolution.* Boston: Extending Horizons Books.

Kuhn, T. S. (1970). *The structure of scientific revolutions* (2nd ed.). Chicago: University of Chicago Press.

Kung, H. (1981). *Does God exist? An answer for today.* New York: Vintage.

Kurtz, L. F. (1997). *Self-help and support group: A handbook for practitioners.* Thousand Oaks, Calif.: Sage Publications.

Kurtz, L. F., & Chambon, A. (1987). Comparison of self help groups for mental health. *Health and Social Work, 12*(4), 275-283.

Lamb, H. R. (1986). Some reflections on treating schizophrenics. *Archives of General Psychiatry, 43,* 1007-1011.

Landeen, J., Pawlick, J., Woodside, H., Kirkpatrick, H., & Byrne, C. (2000). Hope, quality of Life, and symptom severity in individuals with Schizophrenia. *Psychiatric Rehabilitation Journal, 23*(4), 364-369.

Lannert, J. (1991). Resistance and countertransference issues with spiritual and religious clients. *Journal of Humanistic Psychology, 31*(4), 68-76.

Larson, D. B., Sherrill, K. A., Lyons, J. S., et al (1992). Association between dimensions of religious commitment and mental health reported in the American Journal of Psychiatry and the Archives of General Psychiatry: 1978 through 1989. *American Journal of Psychiatry, 149*, 557-559.

Lea, G. (1982). Religion, mental health and clinical issues. *Journal of Religion and Health, 21,* 336-351.

Lee, P. W. H., Lieh-Mak, F., Yu, K. K., & Spinks, J. A. (1993). Coping strategies of schizophrenic patients and their relationship to outcome. *British Journal of Psychiatry, 163*, 177-182.

Leiby, J. (1985). The moral foundations of social welfare and social work. *Social Work, 30*, 323-330.

Leung J & Arthur D G (2004) Clients and facilitators' experiences of participating in a Hong Kong self-help group for people recovering from mental illness. *International Journal of Mental Health Nursing 13,* 232-241.

Leung, M. H. (1994). *The relation between social support and social adjustment of schizophrenia patients in rehabilitation.* Unpublished M.S.W. dissertation. Hong Kong: The Chinese University of Hong Kong.

Levine, M., & Perkins, D. V.(1987). *Principle of community psychology: Perspectives and applications* (pp. 234-257). Oxford University Press: New York.

Levy, L.H. (1976). Self-help Groups: Types and psychological process. *Journal of Applied Behavioral Science, 12*(3), 310-322.

Lewis, G. R. (1984). The attributes of God. In W. A. Elwell (ed.), *Evangelical dictionary of theology* (pp. 196-200). Grand Rapids, Mich : Baker.

Lewis, K.N., & Lewis, D. A. (1985). Impact of religious affiliation of therapists' judgements of patients. *Journal of Consulting and Clinical Psychology, 53,* 926-32.

Liddon, S. C. (1989). *The dual brain, religion, and the unconscious.* Buffalo, NY: Prometheus Books.

Lieberman, M. A. (1990). A group therapist perspective on self-help groups. *International Journal of Group Psychotherapy, 40*(3), 251–278.

Lieberman, M. A., Borman, L. D., & Associates. (1979). *Self help groups for coping with crisis: Origins, members, processes and impact.* San Francisco: Jossey-Fass.

Lieberman, M. A., & Videka-Sherman, L. (1986), The impact of self-help groups on the mental health of widows and widowers. *American Journal of Orthopsychiatry, 56,* 435-449.

Lindgren, K. L., & Coursey, R. D. (1995). Spirituality and serious mental illness: A two-part study. *Psychosocial Rehabilitation Journal, 18*(3), 93-111.

London, P. (1986). *The modes and morals of psychotherapy.* New York: Holt, Rinehart & Winston.

Lowenberg, J.S. (1989). *Caring and responsibility: The crossroads between holistic practice and traditional medicine.* Philadelphia: University of Pennsylvania Press.

LUK A & Shek D T L (2006a) Changes in Chinese discharged chronic mental patients attending a psychiatric rehabilitation program with holistic care elements: A quasi-experimental study. *TSW Holistic Health & Medicine 1, 71-83. DOI 10.1100/tswhhm.2006.26*

LUK A & Shek D T L (2006b) Perceived personal changes in Chinese ex-mental patients attending a holistic psychiatric rehabilitation program. *Social behaviour and Personality 34,* 939-954.

LUK A & Shek D T L (2008) The experiences and perceived changes of Chinese ex-mental patients attending a holistic psychiatric rehabilitation programme: A qualitative study. *Journal of Psychiatric and Mental Health Nursing 15*(6), 447-457.

LUK, L. A. (2004). *The changes of ex-mental patients attending a psychiatric rehabilitation program with holistic care.* Unpublished Ph D. dissertation. Hong Kong: The Chinese University of Hong Kong.

LUK, A. (2011). Investigating the long-term effects of a psychiatric rehabilitation program for persons with serious mental illness in the community: A follow up study *Journal of Clinical Nursing, 20* (19/20): 2712-20 doi: 10.1111/j.1365-2702.2010.03622

Lukkarinen, H., & Hentinen, M. (1997). Assessment of quality of life with the Nottingham Health Profile among patients with coronary heart disease. *Journal of Advanced Nursing, 26,* 73-84.

Lynaugh, J.E., & Fagin, C.M. (1988). Nursing comes of age. *Image, 20,* 184-190.

Ma, J. L. C. (1986). Mutual aid group as a practice model in working with the family members of psychotic patients. *The Hong Kong Journal of Social Work, 10*(1), 40-46.

Ma, J. L. C. (1992). Social support, mutual aid groups, the mentally ill and their families. *Hong Kong Journal of Mental Health, 21,* 16-27.

Mahoney, A., Pargament, K. I., Tarakeshwar, N., & Swank, A. B. (2001). Religion in the home in the 1980s and 1990s: A meta-analytic review and conceptual analysis of links between religion, marriage, and parenting. *Journal of Family Psychology, 15*(4), 559-596.

Mak, K. Y., & Yip, K.S. (1997). The importance of an effective psychiatric community care service for chronic mental patients in Hong Kong. *Hong Kong Journal of Mental Health, 26,* 28-35.

Mallory, L. (1984). *Leading self-help groups: A guide for training facilitators* (pp. 61-66). New York: Family Service America.

Martin, E.J. (1986). Holistic nursing practice: An idea whose time has come. *Journal of Professional Nursing, 2,* 78, 133.

Martin, J. & Romanowski, P. (1998). *Love beyond life: The healing power of after-death communications.* New York: Bantam Books.

Marty, M. E. (1980). Social service: godly and godless. *Social Service Review, 54*(4), 462-81.

Maslow, A. (1968). *Toward a psychology of being* (2nd ed.). New York: VanNostrand/Reinhold.

Mason, W. A., & Windle, M. (2002). A longitudinal study of the effects of religiosity on adolescent alcohol use and alcohol-related problems. *Journal of Adolescent Research, 17*(4), 346-363.

Masters, K. S., & Bergin, A. E. (1992). Religious orientation and mental health. In J. F. Schumaker (Ed.), *Religion and mental Health* (pp. 221-232). Oxford: Oxford University Press.

Maton, K.I. (1988). Social support, organizational characteristics, psychological well-being and group appraisal in three self-help group populations. *American Journal of Community Psychology, 16*(1), 53-77.

Maton, K. I. (1989). The stress-buffering role of spiritual support: Cross-sectional and prospective investigations. *Journal for the Scientific Study of Religion, 28*(3), 310-322.

Maton, K. I., & Wells, E. A. (1995). Religion as a community resource for well-being: Prevention, healing, and empowerment pathways. *Journal of Social Issues, 51*(2), 177-193.

Matson, F. W. (1971). Humanistic theory: The third revolution in psychology. *The Humanist, 31*(2), 7-11.

McAdoo, H., & Crawford, V. (1991). The black church and family support programs. *Prevention in Human Services, 9,* 193-203.

McCullough, M. E., & Snyder, C. R. (2000). Classical source of human strength: Revisiting an old home and building a new one. *Journal of Social Clinical Psychology. 19,* 1-10.

McGuire, C. (1990). An overview of holistic nursing. *Imprint, 37,* 73-74.

Meadow, M. J. (1986). Current and emerging themes in the psychology of religion. *Journal of Psychology and Christianity, 5,* 56-60.

Meystedt, D. M. (1984). Religion and the rural population: Implications for social work. *Social Casework, 65,* 219-226.

Mezzina R, Borg M, Marin I, Sells D, Topor A & Davidson L (2006) From participation to citizenship: How to regain a role, a status, and a life in the process of recovery. *American Journal of Psychiatric Rehabilitation 9,* 39-61.

Moberg, D. (1979). The development of social indicators of spiritual well-being for quality of life research. In D. Moberg (Ed.), *Spiritual well-being: Sociological perspectives,* Washington, DC: University Press of America.

Mok, B. H. (2001). The effectiveness of self-help groups in a Chinese context. *Social Work with Groups, 24*(2), 69-89.

Mok, E. (1997). Attitudes of Chinese nurse towards self-help groups in Hong Kong. *Asian Journal of Nursing Studies, 3*(1), 23-29.

Mok, E. (1998). *A model of empowerment for Hong Kong Chinese cancer patients and the role of the self-help groups in the empowering process.* Hong Kong: Hong Kong Polytechnic University. Unpublished PhD. Thesis.

Muffler, J., Langrod, J., & Larson, D. (1995). There is a balm in Gilead: Religion and substance abuse treatment. In Lowinson, J. H., Ruiz, P., Millman, R. B., Langrod, J. G., (Eds.), *Substance abuse: A comprehensive textbook,* 2nd edition. (pp. 584-595). Baltimore, MD: Williams & Wilkins.

Nakhaima, J. M. (1994). Family counseling: the overlooked resource. *Arete, 19*(1), 46-56.

Nathanson, I. G. (1995). Divorce and women's spirituality. *Journal of Divorce and Remarriage, 22*(3/4), 179-188.

Newman, M. (1989). The spirit of nursing. *Holistic Nursing Practice, 3*(3), 6.

Ng, H. Y., & Shek, D. T. L. (2001). Religion and therapy: Religious conversion and the mental health of chronic heroin-addicted persons. *Journal of Religion and Health, 40*(4), 399-410.

O'Brien, M. E. (1982). The heed for spiritual integrity. In H.Yura, & W. B.Walsh (eds.), *Human needs and the nursing process.* Norwalk, Connecticut: Appleton Century Crofts.

O'Brien, P. J. (1992). Social work and spirituality: clarifying the concept for practice. *Spirituality and Social Work Journal, 3*(1), 2-5.

O'Rourke, C.(1997). Exploring spiritual issues of adults with mental illness in group psychotherapy. *Smith College Studies in Social Work, 67*(2), 177-196.

Oi Hip Fellowship (2000). *Annual Report.* Hong Kong: Christian Oi Hip Fellowship Ltd.

Ortiz, L. (1991). Religious issues: The missing link in social work education. *Spirituality and Social Work Journal, 2*(2), 13-18.

Otto, H.A., & Knight, J.W. (1979). *Dimensions in Wholistic Healing New frontiers in the Treatment of the Whole Person* (p.3). Chicago: Nelson-Hall.

Owen, M.J., & Holmes, C.A. (1993).'Holism'in the discourse of nursing. *Journal of Advanced Nursing, 18,* 1688-1695.

Paloutzian, R. F., & Ellison, C. W. (1982). Loneliness, spiritual well-being and the quality of life. In L.A. Peplau, & Perlman, D. (eds.), *Loneliness: A sourcebook of current theory, research and therapy.* New York: John Wiley & Sons.

Pancoast, D., Parker, P., & Froland, C. (1987). *Rediscovery self-help: Its role in social care. USA: SAGE.*

Pargament, K. I. (1997). *The psychology of religion and coping: Theory, researh, practice.* New York: Guilford.

Pargament, K. I., & Brant, C. R. (1998). Religion and coping. In H. G. Koenig (Ed.), *Handbook of religion and mental health.* California: Academic Press.

Pargament, K. I., & Park, C. L. (1995). Merely a defense? The variety of religious means and ends. *Journal of Social Issues, 51,* 13-32.

Parsons, T. (1960). *Structure and Process in Modern Society.* Chicago: Free Press.

Paukert, A. L., Philips, L. L., Cully, J. A., Romero, C., & Stanley, M. A. (2011). Systematic review of the effects of religion-accommodative psychotherapy for depression and anxiety. *Journal of Contemporary Psychotherapy, 41,* 99-108.

Payne, I. R., Bergin, A. E., Bielema, K. A., & Jenkins, P. H. (1991). Review of religion and mental health: Prevention and the enhancement of psychosocial functioning. *Prevention in Human Services, 9,* 11-40.

Pelletier, K. R. (1979). *Holistic Medicine* (p. 93). New York: Delacorte.

Pelletier, K. R. (2000). *The best alternative medicine: What works? what does not?* New York: Simon and Schuster.

Peterson, C. B., Mitchell, J. E., Crow, S. J., Crosby, R. D., & Wonderlich, S. A. (2009). The efficacy of self-help group treatment and therapist-led treatment for binge eating disorder. *American Journal of Psychiatry, 166*(12), 1347-1354.

Pierce, L.L. (2001). Caring and expressions of spirituality by urban caregivers of people with stroke in African American families. *Qualitative health Research, 11,* 339-352.

Pietroni, P.C. (1986). Spiritual interventions in a general practice setting. *Holistic Medicine, 1,* 253-262.

Pilisuk, M., & Minkler, M. (1985, Winter). Social support: economic and political considerations. *Social Policy,* 6-11.

Polich, J. M., Armor, D. J., & Braiker, H. B. (1981). *The course of alcoholism.* New York: Wiley.

Powell, T. J. (1985). Improving the effectiveness of self help. *Social Policy, 16*(2), 22-29.

Powell, T.J. (1990). *Working with self-help.* Silver Spring: NASW Press.

Pownal, M.(1986, February). All in the mind's eye. *Nursing Times, 82*(8), 26.

Prest, L. A., & Keller, J. F. (1993). Spirituality and family therapy: spiritual beliefs, myths, and metaphors. *Journal of Marital and Family Therapy, 19*(2), 137-148.

Puchalski, C. M. (2006). Spirituality and medicine: curricula in medical education. *Journal of Cancer Education, 21*(1), 14-8.

Pullen, L., Modrcin-talbott, M. A., West, W. R., & Muenchen, R. (1999). Spiritual high vs high on spirits: is religiosity related to adolescent alcohol and drug abuse? *Journal of Psychiatric and Mental Health Nursing, 6*, 3-8.

Pumphrey, R. (1977). *Social welfare: History, encyclopedia of social work* (Vol. 2, p. 1446). New York: National Association of Social Workers.

Radin, D. (1997). The conscious universe: The scientific truth of psychic phenomena. New York: HarperCollins.

Raleigh, E. D. H. (1992). Sources of hope in chronic illness. *Oncology Nursing Forum, 19,* 443-448.

Rasic, D., Robinson, J. A., Bolton, J., Bienvenu, O. J., & Sareen, J. (2011). Longitudinal relationships of religious worship attendance and spirituality with major depression, anxiety disorders, and suicidal ideation and attempts: Findings from the Baltimore epidemiologic catchment area study. *Journal of Psychiatric Research, 45,* 848-854.

Reed, P. (1987). Spirituality and well-being in terminally ill hospitalized adults. *Research in Nursing & Health, 10*(5), 335-44.

Relman, A. (1979). Holistic medicine. *New England Journal of Medicine, 300,* 312-313.

Renshaw, J. (1984, April). The power of the will. *Nursing Times, 80*(1), 38.

Richards, P. S., & Bergin, A. E. (1997). *A spiritual strategy.* Washington, DC: American Psychological Association.

Richardson, J. T. E. (1996). Introduction. In J. T. E. Richardson (Ed.), *Handbook of qualitative research methods.* Leicester: BPS Books.

Rieff, P. (1966). *The triumph of the therapeutic* (p. 97). New York: Harper & Row.

Riessman, F. (1976). How does self-help work? *Social Policy, 7*(2), 41-45.

Riessman, F. (1987). Foreward. In T. J. Powell, *Self- help organization and professional practice* (pp. ix-x). Silver Spring, MD: National Association of Social Workers.

Riessman, F., & Gartner, A. (1987). The surgeon general the self-help Ethos. *Social Policy, 18*(2), 23-25.

Robbins, S. P., Canda, E. R., & Chatterjee, P. (1998). *Contemporary human behavior theory: A critical perspective for social work.* Boston: Allyn & Bacon.

Robinson, D. & Henry, S. (1977). *Self-help and health: mutual aid for modern problems.* London: Martin Robertson.

Rogers, M. (1970). *An introduction to the theoretical basis of nursing.* Philadelphia: F. A. Davis.

Rootes, M.S. & Aanes, D.L. (1992). A Conceptual framework for understanding self-help groups. *Hospital and Community Psychiatry, 43*(4), 379-381.

Ross, L.A. (1997). Elderly patients' perceptions of their spiritual needs and care: A pilot study. *Journal of Advanced Nursing, 26*, 710-715.

Ross, L. (2006). Spiritual care in nursing: an overview of the research to date. *Journal of Clinical Nursing, 15*, 852-862.

Rothlis, J. (1984). The effect of a self-help group on feelings of hopelessness and helplessness. *Western Journal of Nursing Research, 6*(2), 157-173.

Rubel, J. A. (1984). The function of self-help groups in recovery from anorexia nervosa and bulimia. *Psychiatric Clinics of North America, 7*(2), 381-394.

Russel, R. (1998). Spirituality and religion in graduate social work education. In E.R. Canda (ed.), *Spirituality and social work: New directions.* Hazleton, PA: Haworth Press.

Russoinova, Z., Wewiorski, N. J., & Cash, D. (2002). Use of alternative health care practices by persons with serious mental illness: Perceived benefits. *American Journal of Public Health, 92,* 1600-1603.

Rutchick, I. E. (1990). Research on practice with groups in health care settings. *Social Work in Health Care, 15*(1), 97-114.

Saleebey, D.(1997). The strengths approach to practice. In D. Saleebey (Ed.), *The strengths perspective* (pp. 49-57). New York: Longman.

Salem, D. A., Seidman, E., & Rappaport, J. (1988). Community treatment of the mentally ill: The promise of mutual-help organizations. *Social Work, 9*(10), 403-408.

Sanua, V. D. (1969). Religion, mental health, and personality: A review of empirical studies. *American Journal of Psychiatry, 125*, 1203-1213.

Sarkis, J. M., & Sklolner, M M.(1987). An analysis of the concept of holism in nursing literature. *Holistic nursing Practice, 2l,* 61-69.

Saudia, T. L., Kinney, M. R., Brown, K. C., & Upirmg-Ward, L. (1991). Health locus of control and helpfulness of prayer. *Heart and Lung, 20,* 60-65.

Scharlack, A. E. & Fuller, T. E. (1994). Coping strategies following thc dcath of an elderly parent. *Journal of Gernotological Social Work. 21 (3/4),* pp. 85-100.

Scherbourne, C.D. (1988). The role of social support and life stress events in use of mental health services. *Social Science and Medicine, 27*(12), 1393-1400.

Schopler, J. H., & Galinsky, M. J. (1981). When groups go wrong. *Social Work, 26,* 424-429.

Schubert, M. A., & Borkman, T. J. (1991). An organizational typology for self-help groups. *American Journal of Community Psychology, 19*(5), 769-787.

Schumaker, J. F. (1992). *Religion and mental health.* New York: Oxford University Press.

Schwartz, G.E., Simon, W. L., & Linda, G. R. (2002). *The afterlife experiments.* New York: Pocket Books.

Segal, S. P., Silverman, C., & Temkin, T. (1993). Empowerment and self-help agency practice for people with mental disabilities. *Social Work, 38*(6), 705-712.

Sermabeikian, P. (1994). Our clients, ourselves: The spiritual perspective and social work practice. *Social Work, 39*, 178-183.

Shafranske, E. P. (1992). Religion and mental health in early life. In J. F. Schumaker (Ed.), *Religion and mental health* (pp. 163-176). New York: Oxford University Press.

Shafranske, E., & Maloney, H. (1990). Clinical psychologists'religious and spiritual orientations and their practice of psychotherapy. *Psychotherapy, 27,* 72-78.

Shanghai College of Traditional Medicine. (1981). (J. O'Connor & D. Bensky, Trans.). *Acupuncture: A Comprehensive Text.* Chicago: Eastland Press.

Shapiro, D. H. (1982). Overview: Clinical and physiological comparison of meditation and other self-control strategies. *American Journal of Psychiatry, 139,* 267-274.

Shealy, C. N. (2000). *The directory of complementary therapies.* Vancouver: New Millennium.

Sheridan, M. J., & Bullis, R. K. (1991). Practitioners'views on religion and spirituality: A qualitative study. *Spirituality and Social Work Journal, 2*(2), 2-10.

Sheridan, M.J., Bullis, R. K., Adcock, C. R., Berlin, S. D. & Miller, P. C. (1992). Practitioners'personal and professional attitudes and behaviors toward religion and spirituality: Issues for education and practice. *Journal of Social Work Education, 28,* (2),190-203.

Sheridan, M. J., Wilmer, C. M., & Atcheson, L. (1994). Inclusion of content on religion and spirituality in the social work curriculum: A study of faculty views. *Journal of Social Work Education, 30,* 363-376.

Shih, F. J., Gau, M. L., Mao, H. C., Chen, C. H., & Lo, C. H. K. (2001). Empirical validation of a teaching course on spiritual care in Taiwan. *Journal of Advanced Nursing, 36*(3), 333-346.

Shulman, L, & Gitterman, A. (1994). The life model, mutual aid, oppression, and mediating functions. In A. Gitterman, & L. Shulman (Eds.), *Mutual aid groups, vulnerable populations, and the life cycle* (pp. 3-28). New York: Columbia Uni. Press.

Sicher, F., Targ. E., Moore, D. & Smith, H. S. (1998). A randomized double blind study of the effect of distant healing in a population with advanced AIDS: Report of a small scale study. *Western Journal of Medicine, 169,* 356-63.

Siporin, M. (1982). Moral philosophy in social work today. *Social Service Review, 56,* 516-538.

Siporin, M. (1985). Current social work perspectives on clinical practice. *Clinical Social Work Journal, 13,* 198-217.

Siporin, M. (1986). Contribution of religious values to social work and the law. *Social Thought, 12*(4), 35-50.

Sistler, A., & Washington, K. S. (1999). Serenity for African American caregivers. *Social Work with Groups, 22*(1), 49-62.

Skinner, B. F. (1977). A humanist alternative to AA's twelve steps. *The Humanist,* July/August, 5.

Smith, D.H. (1996). Support groups and Psychiatry. *Canadian Journal of Psychiatry, 41*(2), 128.

Smokowski, P. R., Rose, S. D., & Bacallao, M. L. (2001). Damaging experiences in therapeutic groups: How vulnerable consumers become group casualties. *Small Group Research, 32*(2), 223-251.

Smuts, J. C. (1926). *Holism and Evolution*. New York: Macmillan.

Socken, K. & Carson, V. (1987). Responding to the spiritual needs of the chronically ill. *Nursing Clinics of North America, 22* (3), 603-611.

Sperry, R. W. (1988). Psychology's mentalist paradigm and the religion/science tension. *American Psychologist, 43*, 607-613.

Spiegel, D. (1993). *Living beyond limits: new hope and help for facing life-threatening illness.* New York: Times Books.

Spilda, B., & Werme, P. (1971). Religion and mental disorder: A critical review and theoretical perspective. In M. P. Strommen (Ed.), *Research on religious development: A comprehensive handbook.* A project of the Religious Education Association, New York: Hawthorn Books.

St. Stephen's Society (1997). *Help mobile.* (Promotion Pamphlet), St. Stephen's Society.

Stallwood, J. & Stoll, R. (1975). Spiritual dimension of nursing practice. In Beland, I.L., Passos, J. Y. (eds.), *Clinical Nursing* (3rd ed.). New York: Macmillan.

Stark, R. (1971). Psychopathology and religious commitment. *Review of religious research, 12*, 165-176.

Staudt, M., Howard, M. O., & Drake, B. (2001). The operationalization, implementation, and effectiveness of the strengths perspective: A review of empirical studies. *Journal of Social Service Research, 27*(3), 1-21.

Stewart, M. J. (1990). Professional interface with mutual-aid self-help groups: A review. *Social Science in Medicine, 31*(10), 1143-1158.

Stinnett, N. (1979). Strengthening families. *Family Perspective, 13*, 3-9.

Strayhorn, J. M., Weidman, C. S., & Larson, D. (1990). A measure of religiousness, and its relation to parent and child mental health variables. *Journal of Community Psychology, 18*, 34-43.

Strohl, J. E. (1998). Transpersonalism: Ego meets soul. *Journal of Counseling and Development, 76*, 397-403.

Stuart G W & Laraia M T (2005) *Principles and Practice of Psychiatric Nursing.* 8th edn. Mosby, St. Louis, p242.

Strupp, H. H., Hadley, S. W., & Gomes-Schwartz, B. (1977). *Psychotherapy for better or worse: An analysis of the problem of negative effects.* New York: Aronson.

Stux, G., & Pomeranz, B. (1987). *Acupuncture text-book and atlas.* New York: Springer-Verlag.

Sullivan, W. P. (1993). It helps me to be a whole person: The role of spirituality among the mentally challenged. *Psychosocial Rehabilitation Journal, 16,* 125-134.

Sutton, T.D. & Murphy, S.P. (1989). Stressors and patterns of coping in renal transplant patients. *Nursing Research, 38*(1), 46-49.

Talbott, G. D. (1990). Commentary on"Divine intervention and the treatment of chemical dependency", *Journal of Substance Abuse, 2*, 469-471.

Taggart, S. R. (1994). *Living as if.* San Francisco: Jossey-Bass.

Tan, S. Y. (1996). Religion in clinical practice: Implicit and explicit integration. In E. Shafranske (Ed.), *Religion and the clinical practice of psychology* (pp. 365-387). Washington, DC: American Psychological Association.

Tepper, L., Rogers, S. A., Coleman, E. M., & Malony, H. N. (2001). The prevalence of religious coping among persons with persistent mental illness. *Psychiatric Services, 52*(5), 660-665.

Thompson, A. (1990). *Guide to ethical practice in psychotherapy.* New York: Wiley.

Thompson, J. H. (1984). *Spiritual considerations in the prevention, treatment and cure of disease* (p. 8). Boston: Oriel Press.

Thyer, B. A., & Hudson, W. W. (1987). *Progress in Behavioral Social Work.* NY: Haworth.

Tillich, P. (1951). *Systematic theology.* Chicago: University of Chicago Press.

Toseland, R. W, & Siporin, M. (1986). When to recommend group treatment: A review of the clinical and research literature. *International Journal of Group Psychotherapy, 36*(2), 171-202.

Toseland, R.W., & Hacker, L. (1982, July). Self-help groups and professional involvement. *Social Work,* 341-347.

Toulmin, S., & Leary, D. E. (1985). The cult of empiricism in psychology and beyond. In S. Koch & D. E. Leary (Eds.), *A century of psychology as science* (pp. 594-617). New York: McGraw-Hill.

Tournier, P. (1954). *A doctor's case book in the light of the Bible.* London: SCM Press.

Towle, C. (1965). *Common Human Needs.* (rev. ed.) (pp. 6-11). Silver Spring, MD: National Association of Social Workers.

Travelbee, J. (1971). *Interpersonal aspects of nursing.* Philadelphia: F. A. Davis.

Trojan, A. (1989). Benefits of self-help groups: A survey of 232 members from 65 disease-related groups. *Social Science Medicine, 29*(2), 225-232.

Turner, J. G., Clark, A. J., Gauthier, D. K. & Williams, M. (1998). The effect of therapeutic touch on pain and anxiety in burn patients. *Journal of Advanced Nursin, 28,* 10-20.

Twelve Steps and Twelve Traditions. (1952). (p.63). New York: Alcoholics Anonymous.

Uva, J. L. (1991). Alcoholics Anonymous: Medical recovery through a higher power. *Journal of the American Medical Association, 266,* 3064-3067.

Vaillant, G. E. (1983). *The natural history of alcoholism.* Cambridge: Harvard university Press.

Wallace, E. (1983). Freud and religion: A history and reappraisal. In L. Boyer, W. Muensterberger, & S. Grolnick (eds.), *The psychoanalytic study of society,* Vol. 10. Hillsdale: Erlbaum.

Wasserman, H., & Danforth, H. E. (1988). *The human bond: Support groups and mutual aid.* New York: Springer Pub.

Watson, J. (1930). *Introduction to behaviorism.* Chicago: University of Chicago Press.

Watson, M. J. (1985). *Nursing: The philosophy and science of caring.* Denver, CO: Association University Press.

Watson, M. J. (1988). New dimensions of human caring theory. *Nursing Science Quarterly, 1*(4), 175-181.

Weaver, A. J., Samford, J. A., Morgan, V. J., Larson, D. B., Koenig, H. G., & Flannelly, K. J. (2002). A systematic review of research on religion in six primary marriage and family journals: 1995-1999. *American Journal of Family Therapy, 30*(4), 293-309.

Weber, M. (1922). *The Sociology of Religion.* Boston: Beacon Press.

Weber, M. (1930). *The protestant ethic and the spirit of capitalism* (1904), trans. By Talcott Parsons. London: George Allen & Unwin, Ltd.

Werner, E. E., & Smith, R. S. (1982). *Vulnerable, but invincible: A longitudinal study of resilient children and youth.* New York: McGraw-Hill.

Wetzel, M.C. (1991). Depressive and Manic Depressive Association of Tucson, Strengths and Limits: Report by a Bipolar/unipolar Self-Help Group. *Psychological Rehabilitation Journal, 14*(4), 81-85.

Wikler, M. (1986). Pathways to treatment: How Orthodox Jews enter therapy. *Social Casework: The Journal of Contemporary Social Work, 67*(2), 113-18.

Wilber, K., Engler, J., & Brown, D.P. (1986). *Transformation of consciousness.* Boston: Shambala.

Wilson, J. (1978). *Religion in American society: The effective presence.* Englewood Cliffs, NJ: Prentice-Hall.

Wirth, D. P., Richardson, J. T., Eldelman, W. S. & O'Malley, A. C. (1993). Full thickness dermal wounds treated with non-contact therapeutic touch: A replication and extension._*Complementary Therapy Medicine, 1,* 127-32.

Wituk, S., Shepherd, M. D., Slavich, S., Warren, M. L., & Meissen, G. (2000). A topography of self-help groups: An empirical analysis. *Social Work, 45*(2), 157-165.

Wong, D. & Chan, C. (1994). Advocacy on self-help for patients with chronic illness: The Hong Kong experience. In F. Lavoie, T.Borkman, & B. Gidron, (Eds.), *Self-help and mutual aid groups* (pp. 117-139). New York: The Haworth Press, Inc.

Wong, K. F. (1994). *Study on patients'self-help group and community.* Community Development Resource Book 1993 & 1994. Hong Kong: The Hong Kong Council of Social Service. (Chinese Text).

Wong, K. P. (1992). *Self-help groups for persons with chronic illness: An implication to community development.* Community Development Resource Book 1991 & 1992. Hong Kong: The Hong Kong Council of Social Service. (Chinese Text).

Wong, P. T. P. (1998). Meaning-centered counseling In P. T. P. Wong, & P. S. Fry (Eds.), *The human quest for meaning: A handbook of psychological research and clinical applications* (pp. 111-140). Mahwah, N.J.: Erlbaum.

Wong, S.Y.E. (1993). *A study of the self-help movement in Hong Kong: Implications for the role and involvement of social workers.* Unpublished master's thesis, University of Hong Kong, Hong Kong.

Woo, S. Y. (1983). The spiritual approach in drug treatment. In L. MacQuarrie (Ed.), *Drug dependence in Hong Kong* (pp. 139-145). Hong Kong: Hong Kong Polytechnic.

Wood, A. W. (1981). *Karl Marx*. London: Routledge & Kegan Paul, Ltd.

World Health Organization. (1946). *Constitution.* Geneva: WHO.

World Health Organization. (1995). *Field trial: WHOQOL-100.* Division of mental health, Geneva: WHO.

World Health Organization. (1997). *Measuring quality of life: The World Health Organization quality of life instruments.* Geneva: Switzerland.

World Health Organization. (1998). *Health promotion glossary.* Geneva: WHO.

World Health Organization. (2003). *WHO definition of palliative care.* http://www.who.int/cancer/palliative/definition

Yahn, G. (1979). Impact of holistic medicine, medical groups and health concepts. *Journal of the American Medical Association, 242,* 2202-2203.

Yalom, I. D. (1970). *The theory and practice of group psychotherapy.* New York: Basic Books.

Yip, K. S. (1992). A brief description of the self help group for mental ex-patients: GROW in Australia, *Hong Kong Journal of Mental Health, 20,* 6-15

Yip, K. S. (1996). A historical review of the community care movement in psychiatric services. *Hong Kong Journal of Psychiatry, 6(1),* 38-44.

Yip, K. S. (1997). An overview of the development of psychiatric rehabilitation services in Hong Kong. *Hong Kong Journal of Psychiatry, 26,* 8-27.

Yiu, L.S.W. & Ng, C.P.Y. (1989). An outlet? Ex-mental patients in a mutual help organization in the community. In C. Chan & A. Yeung (Ed.), *Community Work – the practice of community care* (pp.111-125). Hong Kong: The Hong Kong Social Workers' Association (In Chinese).

Yoak, M., & Chesler, M. (1985). Alternative professional roles in health care delivery: Leadership patterns in self-help groups. *Journal of Applied Behavioral Science, 21*(4), 427-444.

York, G. Y. (1987). Religious-based denial in the NICU: Implications for social work. *Social Work in Health Care, 12*(4), 31-45.

INDEX

D

E

F

G

H

I

J

K

L

M

N

O

P

Q

R

S

T